ashtanga yoga

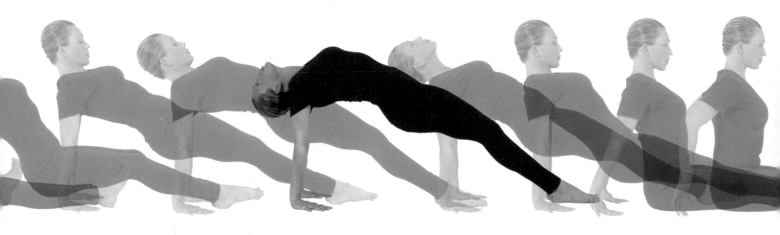

a *flow**motion*™ title

ashtanga yoga

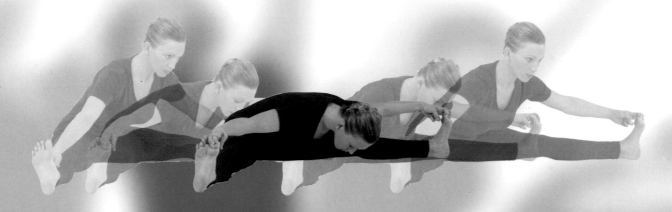

vickie wills

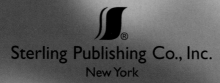

Sterling Publishing Co., Inc.

New York

Created and conceived by
Axis Publishing Limited
8c Accommodation Road
London NW11 8ED
www.axispublishing.co.uk

Creative Director: Siân Keogh
Managing Editor: Brian Burns
Project Designer: Anna Knight
Project Editor: Christopher Norris
Production Manager: Sue Bayliss
Photographer: Mike Good

Library of Congress Cataloging-in-Publication
Data Available

10 9 8 7 6 5 4 3 2 1

Published in 2002 by Sterling Publishing Co., Inc.
387 Park Avenue South, New York, NY 10016
Text and images © Axis Publishing Limited 2002
Distributed in Canada by Sterling Publishing
C/o Canadian Manda Group,
One Atlantic Avenue, Suite 105
Toronto, Ontario, M6K 3E7, Canada

Separation by
United Graphics Pte Limited
Printed and bound by
Star Standard (Pte) Limited

Sterling ISBN 0–8069–9382–0

a *flowmotion*™ title

ashtanga yoga

contents

introduction

Yoga is the union of mind and body. We achieve this union through breath. The beauty of yoga is that when practiced with commitment and enthusiasm it enriches your life in so many different ways. It will lead you to a healthier body inside and out, a calmer mind and a more stress-free life.

Yoga is of course, in origin, a Hindu belief system aiming at the mystical union of the self with the supreme being. However, you do not have to have any specific belief system to practise it. Yoga works more like a science, focusing on the breath, body and mind, bringing them all together through physical and mental exercises. Nor do you have to eat a special diet or drink herbal teas. You do not even need a peace-and-love philosophy of life, though you might find that comes naturally with the tranquility achieved through Yoga. All that you really need is a desire to learn and practice.

People begin to practice yoga for many different reasons. The positive health benefits include more restful sleep, increased energy levels, better concentration, improved muscle tone, greater flexibility, stress relief, and an overall feeling of emotional and physical wellbeing.

Looking after the physical health of our bodies while calming our minds in this ever more frantic world we now live in can only be a step forward to a more healthy and enjoyable life.

You may already know that there are many different forms of yoga. Hatha yoga, Iyengar yoga, and Sivananda yoga—to name just a few. In essence, they are all just different roads to the same place. The style of yoga described in this book is known as Ashtanga Vinyasa yoga. The main difference between Ashtanga Vinyasa yoga and other styles is that it is much more dynamic and physically demanding as it places greater emphasis on "movement when linking the postures"—the vinyasas.

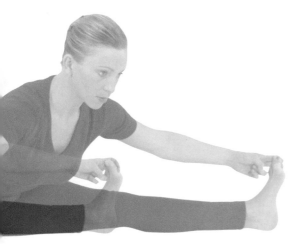

It will take some practice before you should attempt this intense wide-leg forward bend

ASHTANGA VINYASA YOGA

The Ashtanga Vinyasa yoga system that is now practiced originates from the yoga sutras of patanjali, devised in about 200 BC. These sutras were later translated by Krisnamaracharya into a more accessible system that could be taught and practiced by a much wider audience. Shri K Pathabi Jois, one of Krisnamaracharya's main students, continues to teach the Ashtanga Vinyasa yoga system today and is considered to be the guru of Ashtanga yoga.

- **ashta**—eight

- **anga**—limb

- **yoga**—union

- **vinyasa**—flow, the synchronized movement of the body and breath to create a flowing sequence.

the eight limbs of ashtanga

1 **yama**—attitudes
2 **niyama**—physical disciplines
3 **asana**—postures
4 **pranayama**—breathing
5 **pratyahara**—withdrawal of senses
6 **dharana**—concentration
7 **dhyana**—meditation
8 **samhadi**—absorption

YAMA HAS FIVE ASPECTS

ahimsa—non-violence
satya—honesty
asteya—no stealing, openness
bhramacharya—focus
aparigraha—non-possessiveness

NIYAMA ALSO HAS FIVE ASPECTS

saucca—commitment
samtosa—willingness
tapas—enthusiasm
svadyaya—self inquiry
ishvarapranidhana—devotion

YAMA

AHIMSA: Not roughly pushing our way through or past a tight, weak muscle or area of our body. Be gentle, and respect the limitations our bodies and minds are experiencing.

SATYA: Being honest with ourselves while practicing. If we know that we can straighten our leg in a posture, then we should do so, but we should not try to do something we know we are not ready for.

ASTEYA: Not trying to get more from our practice or any one posture that is not naturally there to be gained. Be open to what you can find and experience.

BHRAMACHARYA: Staying focused and not wasting energy by fidgeting and letting your mind wander away from your aim of practicing the posture.

APARIGRAHA: Not being possessive about our achievements in the postures. Just because we got so far in a posture during our previous practice does not mean it will be the same today.

NIYAMA

SAUCCA: We must practice each time with total commitment and no half measures. We must commit ourselves, our minds, and bodies, to practice without any doubts or hesitations.

SAMTOSA: We must practice willingly and happily without resentment and because we want to do so, not because we feel we have to.

TAPAS: We must practice with a burning desire and enthusiasm for what we are doing.

SVADYAYA: We must understand and accept that our practice—if not to begin with—will become a time of self-inquiry, a mirror of ourselves.

ISHVARAPRANIDHANA: We must practice with kindness and humility, being grateful for who we are and be devoted to whatever we do.

ASANA: The physical postures must be practiced with breath awareness and synchronicity. To practice these postures without yama, niyama, and pranayama (and with the Bhandas engaged, see pages 10–11) is more stretching than other yoga styles.

PRANAYAMA: Breathing exercises are used to refine the breath and increase our ability to breathe more freely. Advanced pranayama exercises should only be practiced when you have a deeper understanding of asana and only under the guidance of an experienced teacher.

PRATYAHARA: Learning to internalize the senses by constantly bringing the mind back to the breath when it gets distracted by other thoughts, sounds, movements, or physical distractions within the body. Learning to let these things happen, without attaching any thoughts to them, so that they immediately pass on, as the focus stays with the breath.

DHARANA: Achieving a deep state of pratyahara. When your mind is focused on the breath and is no longer distracted by external forces, you can then begin to achieve a deep level of concentration.

DHYANA: Meditation that has moved on, past concentration. The mind has become still, tranquil and unhindered by conscious thought.

SAMHADI: This can be described as many things: total absorption; a pure state of joy to be at one with God; a true state of being. To put one specific definition to it, I feel, would be wrong. Each person, I believe, experiences it in a different way.

bhandas

BHANDAS: LOCK, SEAL The Bhandas are used to direct the energy created by the breath. Essential to the practice of Ashtanga yoga are the three Bhandas:

MULA BHANDA Root lock, located in the very lower abdomen towards the perineum.

UDDIYANA BHANDA Upward flying, diaphragm lock, located in the middle section of the torso where the abdomen finishes and the ribs start.

JALANDARA BHANDA Throat lock, located in the throat.

UJJAYI PRANAYAMA Victorious breath: the breathing technique that is used in Ashtanga Yoga. It creates an internal heat within the body and helps to focus the mind. Developing control of the Bhandas together with Ujjayi pranayama gives stability and energy to the postures, keeping your practice alive.

PRACTISING MULA BHANDA As you exhale, start to gently suck your lower abdomen between the belly button and the pelvic floor, in and up. Feeling the perineum lifting slightly, gently increase that lift. As you do this, you will notice your anus beginning to tighten slightly.

PRACTICING UDDIYANA BHANDA Uddiyana bhanda can be found at the very end of your exhalation when your lungs are empty. Just before you inhale, lift the lower abdomen and stomach in and up as if under the ribcage. This directs the inhalation upwards to fill the lungs as the ribs open sideways using the intercostal muscles. Begin to expand the ribs, allowing the lungs to take in more air.

PRACTICING JALANDARA BHANDA This involves partially closing the glottis as if you were about to swallow. It is applied to create Ujjayi pranayama, so the two happen alongside each other.

Inhalation with Bhandas—note how the diaphragm lock tightens the line of the torso

PRACTICING UJJAYI PRANAYAMA Activate Jalandara bhanda by partially closing the glottis. As you inhale, keeping the mouth closed and breathing softly through the nose, filter the breath down through the back of the throat. You should be able to feel the breath in your throat. This creates a soft, sibulent sound. Exhale softly through the nose again. Breathing in this way creates an internal heat and the rhythm to which you practice. Trying to keep the breath soft, fluid, and even. Listening to your breath and not overlooking it or pushing it when it becomes restricted will help you to practice safely and keep you free from injury.

The application of Uddiyana and Jalandara bhanda during the asana practice, and in relation to Ujjayi pranayama, is very subtle. Full Uddiyana and Jalandara bhandas are practiced during pranayama.

All three Bhandas must be engaged throughout your practice. They create stability and help create a strong

When inhaling without Bhandas, the line of the torso is looser as seen here

foundation for your practice. They are essential to the practice of Ashtanga yoga, as is Ujjayi pranayama.

The breath is the tool with which you unite the body and mind. The Bhandas are used to hold and direct the "pranic energy" created by the breath.

DRISHTI—GAZE POINTS Within each posture there is a focal point towards which you direct your gaze. The gaze points are used to focus your energy inwards and to stay centered. These are also considered essential to the practice of Ashtanga yoga—although I feel, to begin with, learning the correct drishti for each posture can sometimes create tension in the body and confusion in the mind. Be patient; once you have become more familiar with the postures and your practice has become more stable, you will have a stronger foundation from which to learn the correct drishtis alongside the postures from your teacher. Letting the gaze fall naturally as a result of the position of the head and keeping a soft focus will be more beneficial to begin with.

posture and alignment

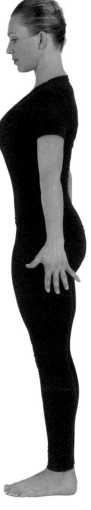

Correct posture is essential to achieve maximum benefit from the yoga postures. This will also protect you from immediate injury and prevent unnecessary tension accumulating from continued bad postural alignment.

FEET Spread the weight evenly between both feet. "Ground" the four corners of each foot from the ball of the big toe across the ball of the foot to the little toe. Ground from the inner heel across to the outer heel. Keep the toes long and relaxed, creating space between each toe.

KNEES AND THIGHS The thigh muscles should be kept engaged. Suck the thigh muscles up and around the thigh bone, lifting the kneecap. Avoid pushing the kneecap back as this will only encourage hyperextension in the back of the knee and bring undue pressure into the knee joint.

In the correct posture, as seen here, body weight is spread evenly between both feet, the lower back is relaxed, and the pelvis kept level

LOWER BACK, PELVIS, HIPS, AND BUTTOCKS The pelvis should be kept level, not tucking under and clenching the buttocks or rolling back with the bottom sticking out. The lower back should be kept relaxed, allowing for the natural curve of the spine. This is supported by keeping the front hip bones gently lifting and the buttock muscles relaxed.

THE THIGH MUSCLES

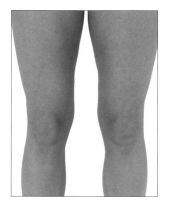 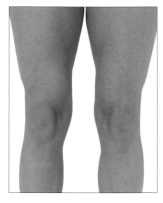

Relaxed thighs, as shown above, are not the correct posture for Ashtanga

Engaged thighs, with the muscles up and around the thigh bone, are the correct posture

THE TORSO The Bhandas should be engaged while the external abdominal muscles are kept long and soft.

SHOULDERS, ARMS, AND HANDS Shoulders should be relaxed and away from the ears. Shoulder blades should be kept moving down the back. The chest and back should be kept open and broad. Wrists should be in line with the forearms, palms open, and fingers long.

HEAD AND NECK The back of the neck should be kept in line with the spine by keeping the chin lowered slightly. The facial muscles should be kept passive and soft. Try not to frown or grimace, even when the postures become more challenging.

POSTURE CHECKLIST

Beginners and more advanced students alike may find it helpful to do a quick mental checklist. When you have moved into a posture:

- Ground the feet
- Engage the thighs
- Align the pelvis
- Engage the Bhandas
- Relax the shoulders
- Engage the arms
- Keep your neck in line with your spine

Eventually this checklist should not be necessary as these things will happen naturally and will not need to be thought of separately.

asanas and posture

If you find any of the postures in this book too challenging or painful, or if they create a sense of panic when attempting them, stop doing them. Discuss the problems you are having with a teacher. This book should be used as an aid to your practice and help you gain a better understanding of the postures. It is not and should never be used as a replacement for learning from a teacher.

GETTING READY TO PRACTICE

Decide how long you wish to practice for. If you are not on a tight schedule, practice until you decide you want to finish—letting your practice come to a natural end. Turn off the phone. Stopping to answer the phone will disrupt the flow of energy you have created during your practice. Make sure there are no draughts in the space you will be practicing in as cold air on warm muscles is likely to cause muscle strain. Take off jewellery such as watches, charms, and so on. They will only get in the way. Wear clothes that don't restrict your movement either because they are too tight or too baggy. Try to practice on an empty stomach or leave at least two hours after a light meal.

During your practice it is important that you stay focussed, trying not to let your mind wander. Be constantly aware of what your body and mind are doing. Remember everything you are doing is a new experience for your mind as well as all the muscles, ligaments, and tendons that you will use to articulate the postures. Your practice is not a competition, it is not a "no pain, no gain" workout or a feel-the-burn cardio class. Your yoga practice should be approached with care and understanding of your body's limitations. Take yourself to the edge where all your muscles are working to support the posture but there is no pain or extreme tension anywhere in the body. Use your breath to relax and you will find that your edge will move, allowing you to go deeper into the posture with ease and comfort. Look after your body and your mind, and in turn they will look after you.

go with the flow

The special *Flowmotion* images used in this book have been created to ensure you see the whole of each exercise—not just selected highlights. Each exercise is labelled suitable for advanced beginners, intermediate, or advanced students by a coloured tab above the title. The captions along the bottom of the images provide additional information to help you perform the exercises confidently. Below this, another layer of information includes instructions for breathing and symbols indicating when to hold a position. The order the exercises are shown in the book is a suggested sequence only. Beginners should pick out suitable exercises, while intermediate and advanced practitioners can create their own programme.

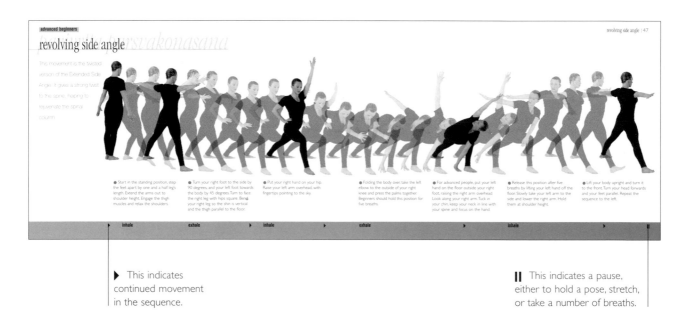

▶ This indicates continued movement in the sequence.

❚❚ This indicates a pause, either to hold a pose, stretch, or take a number of breaths.

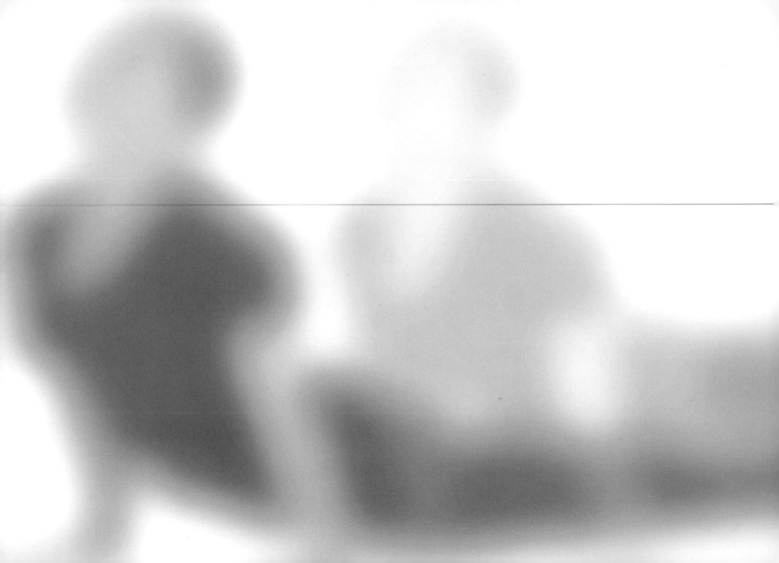

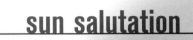

sun salutation

sun salutation "a"

surya namaskara "a"

This movement is one of two
types of greeting to the Sun
god, Surya. Traditionally,
these Salutations are
practiced in the morning,
at the start of your daily
yoga session.

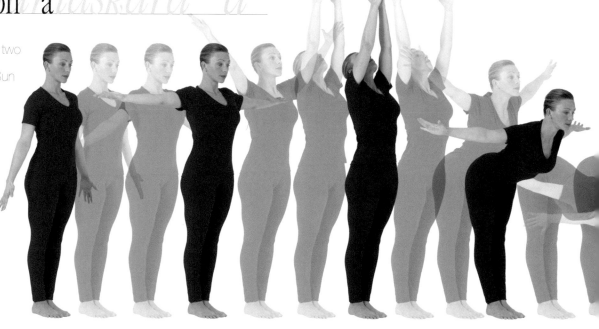

● Stand with feet together and toe
joints and ankles touching. Engage the
thighs and the Bhandas. Relax your
shoulders and extend your arms by
your side.

● Rotate your arms out to the sides,
turning the palms so that they face
outward. Take the arms up above
your head, then gently tip back your
head to look upward. Turn the palms
inward and press them together.

● Bend forward from the hips, as you
bring your arms out and down to the
sides. Keeping your torso lengthened,
take your chest toward your knees so
that your ribs move away from your
hips.

▶ **inhale**   ▶ **exhale**   ▶

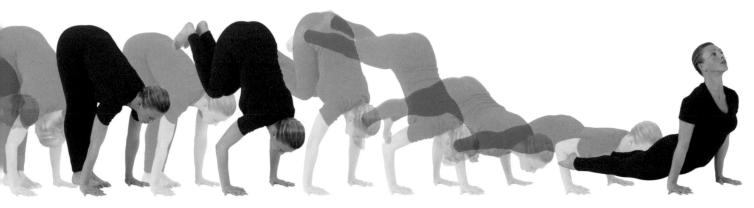

● Place your hands on the floor, or on your legs, if this is more comfortable. Pushing into your hands, lift the chest and extend your torso. Focus the eyes forward, beyond your hands.

● Bending your knees if necessary, transfer your body weight from the feet to the hands. Lift the hips high and jump back onto the balls of your feet, keeping your chest open and elbows in.

● Roll your feet over your toes, taking the chest forward at the same time.

● Straighten your arms, lift up the chest and look up toward the sky. Press your feet into the floor so that your knees come off the floor. This is the Upward Dog position. This sequence continues on the next page.

sun salutation "a"

surya namaskara "a"

When practicing the sun Salutations, keep the movements smooth and graceful—imagine you are waking your body gradually and gently at the start of a new day.

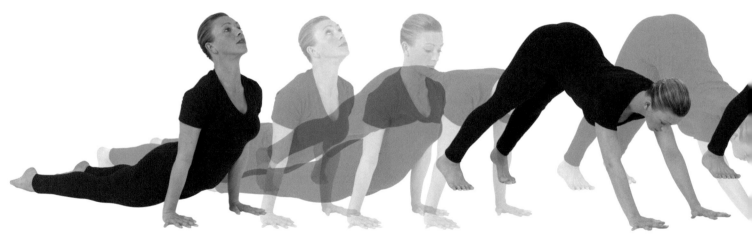

● Your spine, thighs, and legs should be fully extended. Focus on keeping your chest open with your head up and slightly back.

● Tuck in your chin and look down toward the floor in between your hands.

● Keeping your arms and legs straight, roll your feet back over the toes, lifting your bottom high into the air.

● Pushing against the floor with the palms of your hands. Aim to press your heels into the floor and point your buttocks upward to create an inverted "V"-shape.

exhale ▶ ▶ ▶

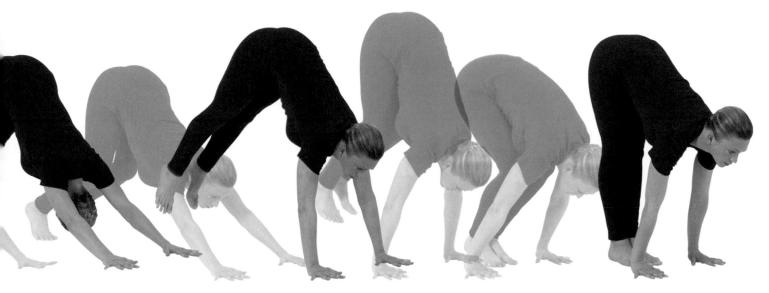

● Hold this position, the Downward Dog, for five breaths. Focus completely on the breathing.

● Shift your body weight onto the balls of your feet, raising your heels off the ground. Bend your knees and focus your eyes on a point beyond your hands at the end of your exhalation.

● Push your feet away from the ground, carrying your hips high as you jump. Bring your feet to land inside the outstretched arms. Keep your torso extended with head and chest lifted.

● Move your ribs away from your hips. The soles of the feet and palms of your hands should be pressed firmly against the floor. This sequence continues on the next page.

❙❙　▶　**inhale**　▶

sun salutation "a"

surya namaskara "a"

The final part of this movement brings you back to the standing position, from where you can repeat the Salutation several times over to ensure your body is sufficiently warmed up. However, this is not just a warm-up routine, but an essential part of your yoga practice.

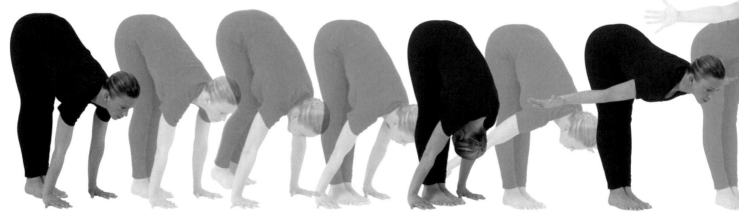

● Still holding the body in its folded position, raise your head slightly to feel a stretch along the spine. Bring the hips forward a little to help keep the legs at right angles to the ground.

● Release the stretch in the spine and slowly bring your head forward, tucking the chin into your chest.

● Take the chest toward your knees, sliding your hands back along the ground until they are level with your feet. Keep your arms fully extended.

● Lift your hands off the floor and take your arms out to the sides, with palms facing upward. Slowly unfurl the body, taking the head and chest forward. Keep your legs straight and feet firmly pressed on the ground.

exhale ▶ **inhale** ▶

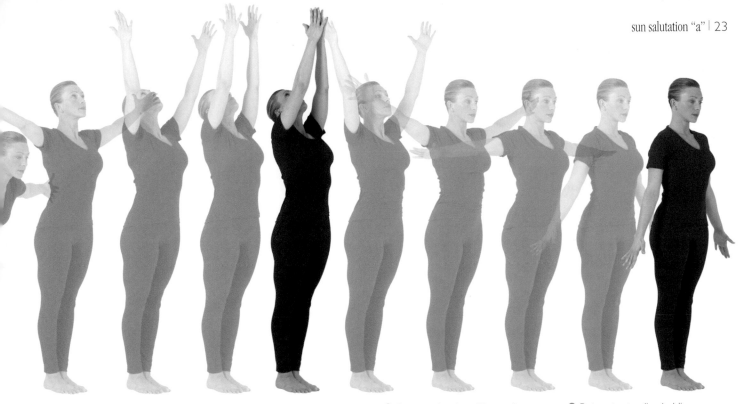

● Rotate the arms so that your palms face forward and continue lifting them toward the sky. Raise your torso upward until the spine is fully extended, and let your gaze follow your arms upward.

● When the arms are fully extended above your head, press the palms together. Keep your gaze fixed on your hands as you do this.

● Part your hands and lower the arms to your sides. Lower your head and focus your eyes forward.

● Return to standing, holding your head upright, back straight, and chest open. Repeat the whole sequence three to five times.

▶   exhale   ▶   ‖

sun salutation "b"
surya namaskara "b"

This second version of the Sun Salutation movement also provides the body with a wake-up that focuses on awakening every part of the body.

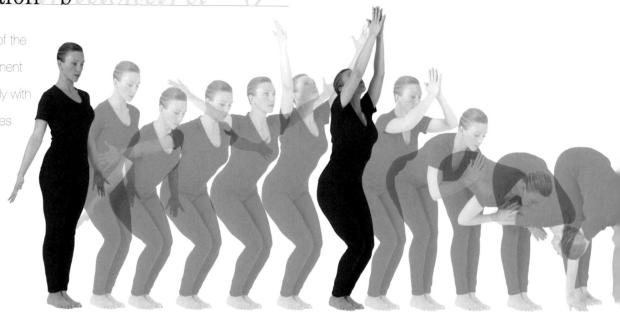

● Start by standing with feet together and toe joints and ankles touching. Engage the thighs and the Bhandas. Relax your shoulders and extend your arms by your sides.

● Rotate your arms out to the sides, with palms facing outward. At the same time, bend your knees and let your bottom drop over the heels. Take the arms up above your head and press the palms together.

● Fold forward from the hips, move the chest toward your knees. Release your hands to touch the floor. Tuck your chin into the chest.

▶ **inhale** ▶ **exhale** ▶

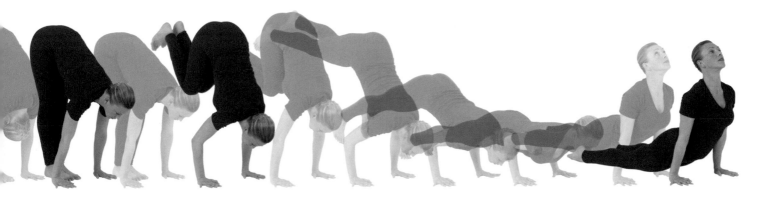

● Press your hands into the floor, lift the chest, extend the torso and look forwards.

● Bending your knees if necessary, transfer your body weight from the feet to the hands. Lift the hips high and jump back onto the balls of your feet, keeping your chest open and elbows in.

● Roll your feet over your toes, taking the chest forward at the same time.

● Straighten your arms, lift up the chest, and look up toward the sky. Press your feet into the floor so that your knees come off the floor. This is Upward Dog. The sequence continues on the next page.

| inhale | exhale ▶ | inhale ▶ | inhale | 11 |

sun salutation "b"

Except where indicated otherwise, focus on keeping an alignment between your head, neck, and spine throughout this sequence. This will help you to practice safely and will also add some stability to the entire Salutation. Perform the Salutation gradually and carefully.

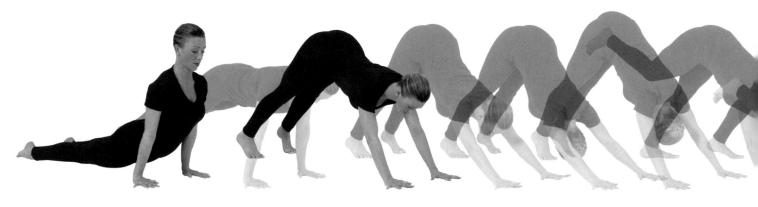

● Hold your head upright, but look downward with your eyes, still pushing your body away from the ground.

● Keeping your arms and legs straight, roll your feet back over the toes, lifting your bottom high into the air.

● Push against the floor with the palms of your hands. Aim to press your heels into the floor and point your buttocks upward to create an inverted "V"-shape.

● Raise your heels off the ground. Turn your left heel in slightly and raise your right foot off the ground.

exhale ▶   ▶ inhale   ▶

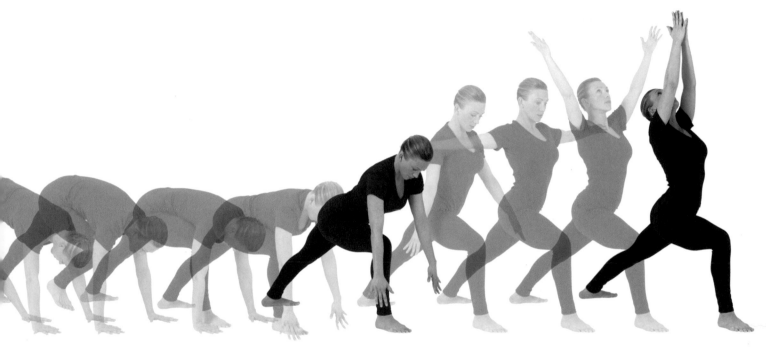

● Bend your right leg and push the knee forward. Lift your chest away from the thighs and raise your head to face the ground.

● Step forward with your right leg, and place the foot on the ground to the inside of your right arm. Raise your hands onto the fingertips and let your feet take the body weight.

● Raise your body into the upright position. Extend the arms up, taking them out to the sides. Keep your gaze downward until the arms are level with your shoulders.

● Rotate the arms so that the palms face upward, and lift them above the head until the palms come together. Keep your back upright, with hips and chest lifted. Tilt your head back gently and focus on your hands.

▶   inhale   ▶   II

sun salutation "b"

Continue the Sun Salutation steadily and as gracefully as possible. In this section, focus on feeling your body weight evenly distributed between the hands and feet when you are on all fours.

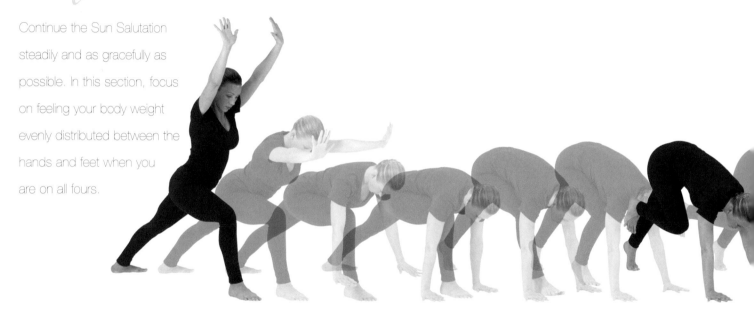

● Release the pose and part your hands. Bring the outstretched arms forward, lowering them them toward the ground. Place the palms face down on either side of your right foot.

● Push forward onto the ball of your left foot, raising the heel. Shift your weight onto your left foot and hands.

● Raise the right foot, bringing the knee into your chest, and then step it back until it is level with your left foot.

exhale ▶ ▶ ▶

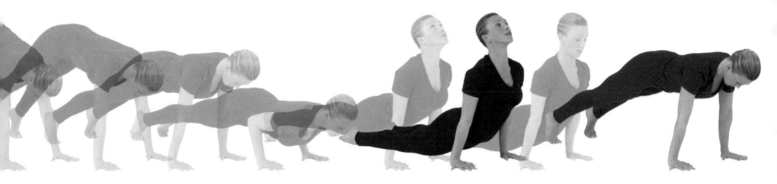

● Keep both heels off the floor and continue pressing down on your palms. Your weight should be evenly distributed between hands and feet. Lower your body until it is parallel with the ground.

● Keep your elbows tucked in and shoulders away from your ears.

● Roll your feet over the toes, taking the chest forward at the same time. Straighten your arms, lift up the chest, and look up toward the sky. This is the Upward Dog position.

● Keeping your arms and legs straight, lift your bottom high into the air. The sequence continues on the next page.

exhale ▶ **inhale** **exhale** ▶

sun salutation "b"

This section includes a complete movement from facing the floor to reaching up to the sky.

This range of movement helps to get the blood flowing throughout the body and effectively

wakes the body up ready for the rest of your yoga routine.

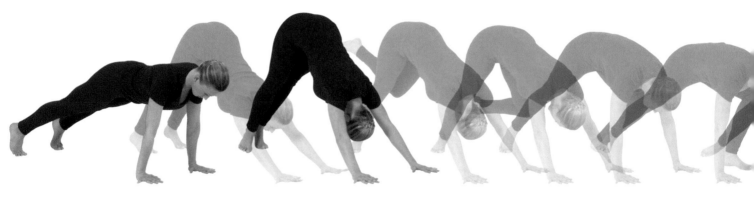

● Push against the floor with the palms of your hands. Aim to press your heels into the floor and point your buttocks upward to create an inverted "V"-shape.

● Raise your heels off the ground. Turn your right heel in slightly and raise your left foot off the ground.

● Bend your left leg and push the knee forward. Lift your chest away from the thighs and raise your head to face the ground.

● Step forward with your left leg, and place the foot on the ground to the inside of your left arm. Raise your hands onto the fingertips and let your feet take the body weight.

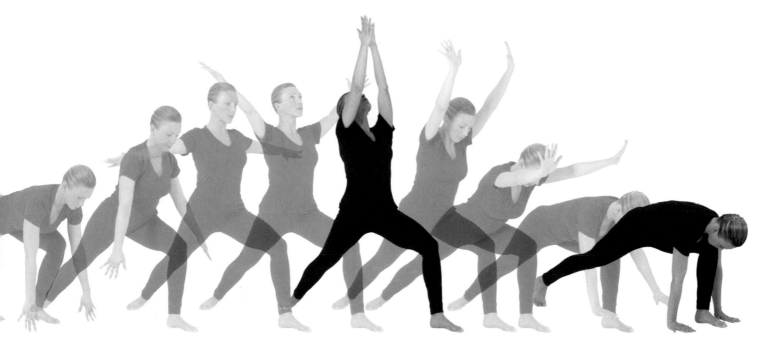

● Raise your body into the upright position. Extend the arms up, taking them out to the sides. Keep your gaze downward until the arms are level with your shoulders.

● Rotate the arms so that the palms face upward, and lift them above the head. Keep your back upright, with hips and chest lifted. Tilt your head back gently and focus on your hands.

● Release the pose and part your hands. Bring the outstretched arms forward, lowering them them toward the ground. Place the palms face down on either side of your left foot.

● Push forward onto the ball of your right foot, raising the heel. Shift your weight onto your right foot and hands. The sequence continues on the next page.

▶ **exhale**

sun salutation "b"

Once again, this movement takes you from facing the floor to reaching for the sky. Both versions of the Salutation provide an all-round wake up for your muscles and circulation. Remember that they are part of your yoga routine, not a separate warm-up routine.

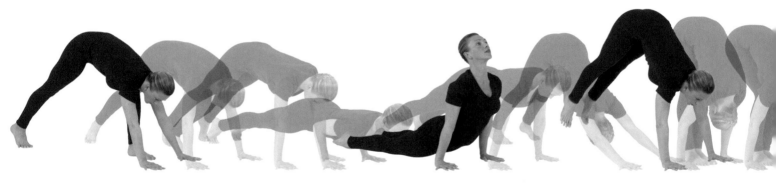

● Raise the right foot, bringing the knee into your chest and then step it back until it is level with your left foot.

● Push against the floor with your hands. Aim to press your heels into the floor and point your buttocks upward to create an inverted "V"-shape. Hold for five breaths.

● At the end of your exhale, bend the knees and look to the hands. Push your feet away from the ground, carrying your hips high as you jump.

● Bring your feet to land inside the outstretched arms. Keep your torso extended with head and chest lifted. Fold forward, keeping the ribs moving away from the hips, and the chest moving toward the knees.

| exhale ▶ | inhale ▶ | exhale ▶ |

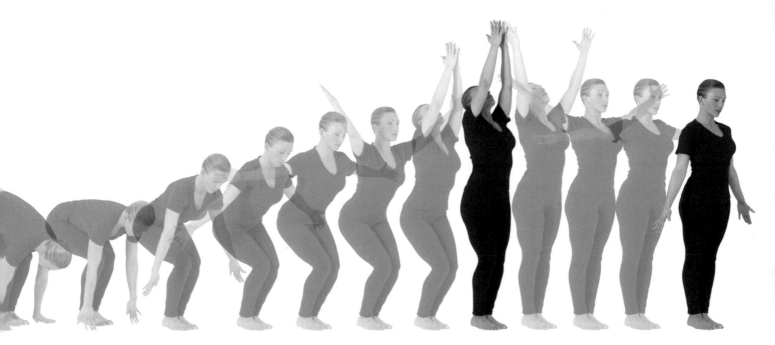

● Still holding the body in its folded position, raise your head slightly to feel a stretch along the spine. Bend at the knees and start to lift the torso away from the thighs as you take the arms overhead, palms together.

● Keep the feet together as you gradually straighten your knees.

● Extend your arms fully above your head, press the palms together and keep your gaze fixed on your hands.

● Move the hands apart and bring them down to your side. Repeat the whole sequence three to five times.

inhale ▶ exhale ‖ ▶ ‖

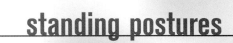

standing postures

hands to toes
padangusthasana

This sequence helps to increase the flex ability in your hamstrings. You may find it easier to bend your knees when holding the toes or feet.

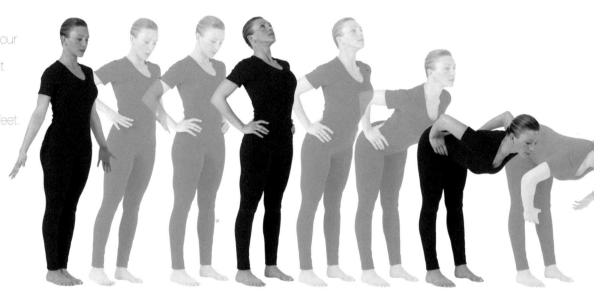

● Start with feet together, back and head held upright, and arms outstretched at the sides. Engage the Bhandas.

● Raise your arms slightly and place your hands on your hips. At the same time, step your feet hip-width apart. Lift your chest and look up toward the ceiling.

● Bend your body forward at the hips, keeping your back straight throughout the movement. Continue moving your chest toward the knees.

inhale ▶ **exhale** ▶

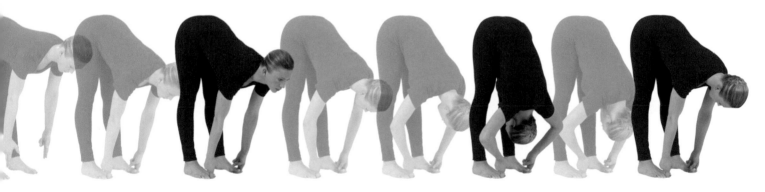

● Form a hook with the first fingers and thumb. Hook the fingers inside and under the big toes.

● Extend your torso, lifting the chest away from the legs and look forward.

● Move your chest closer to the knees and tuck your chin in. Bend your elbows outward and take five breaths. This position is known as hands to toes, or *Padangusthasana*.

● Pull against your feet, lifting the chest upward. Straighten your arms and hold your shoulders away from your ears to feel a stretch. This sequence continues on the next page.

exhale   **inhale**   **exhale**   **inhale**   ▶

hands to feet *padahastasana*

The second part of this movement—Hands to Feet—is the more strenuous

exercise. Stretch from the hips, rather than from the shoulders.

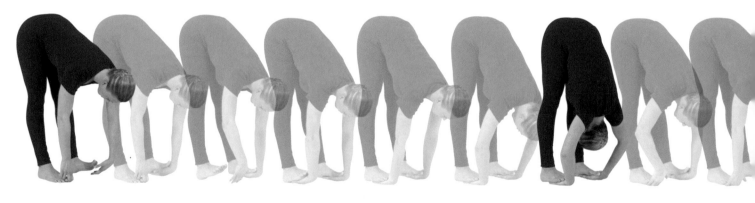

● One foot at a time, lift the sole off the floor and place a hand underneath. Step your foot on top of your hand.

● Increase the fold in the body by moving your chest toward the thighs. Keep your legs straight and let the arms bend at the elbows to allow the head to drop further down.

● Tuck your chin into the chest and fix your gaze on a point between your knees. Hold this pose for five breaths. If this position feels uncomfortable, bend your knees.

● Release the hold and gently ease your hands out from under your feet. Straighten your arms and slowly raise your head so that it faces the floor.

▶   **exhale**   ▶   ▶   **inhale**   ▶

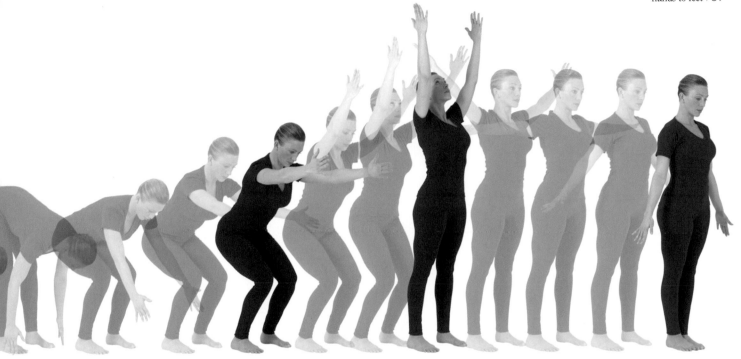

● Bend your knees and drop your bottom toward the heels. Keep your feet firmly on the floor. As you raise your chest away from the thighs, lift your outstretched arms in front of your body.

● Stretch your arms above your head, with palms facing each other. Let your gaze follow your hands until you are looking upward.

● Breathe out as you bring the arms back down to your sides. Bring the head upright and look forward.

● As the arms come down to your sides, step the feet together. Pause a moment before beginning the next sequence.

exhale

extended triangle *utthita trikonasana*

This movement creates an effective side stretch that also continues down the back of the leg. It also strengthens the ankles and thighs.

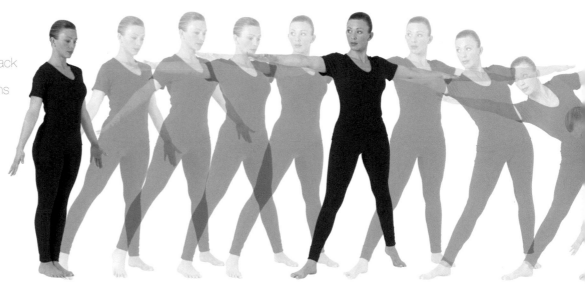

● From the standing position, step your feet apart by one leg's length. Raise your arms up to shoulder height, with palms facing downward. Engage your thigh muscles and relax the shoulders.

● Turn your right foot out to the side by 90 degrees, and turn your left foot to the body by 10 to 15 degrees. Turn your head to the right, so that you are looking along your right arm.

● Engage the thighs and press both feet firmly into the floor to create a stable base for the stretch.

▶ inhale   ▶ exhale   ▶ inhale   ▶

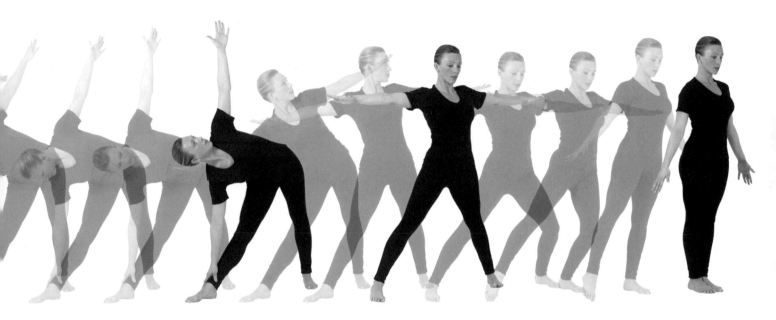

● With your right arm leading, lean the body out over your right leg, bending from the waist. Rest your right hand on your shin.

● Turn your head to the front and then to the left, to look along your left arm which is now pointing upward. Hold this position for five breaths.

● Take your hand away from the shin and slowly raise your body into the upright position, until it is facing forward again. Turn both feet so that the toes are pointing forward.

● From a standing position, repeat the sequence to the left, taking the left hand down to the left shin.

exhale ▶ **inhale** **exhale** ▶ **II**

revolving triangle
pariantta trikonasana

The Revolving Triangle movement is developed from the Extended Triangle on the previous pages. It tones the thigh, stretches the hamstring, and stimulates the spine and back muscles.

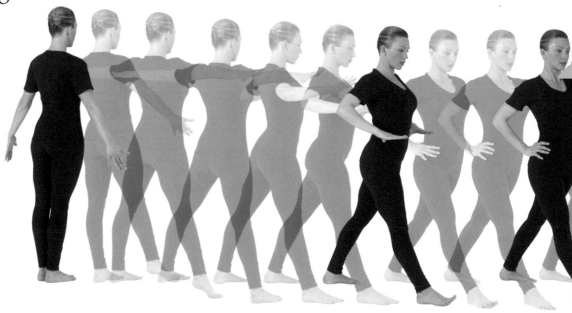

● Start in the standing position, with feet together and arms by your sides. Step your feet apart by one leg's length and slowly raise your arms to shoulder height.

● Bend your arms and place your hands onto the hips. Turn your right foot out to the side by 90 degrees, and turn your left foot inward by 45 degrees. Align your hips with your right leg. Do not let your back arch.

● Reach up with your left arm, keeping your right hand on your hip and your body aligned along your right foot.

inhale ▶ **exhale** ▶ **inhale** ▶

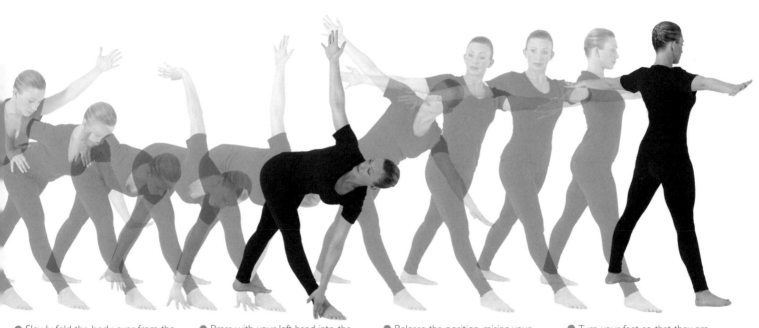

● Slowly fold the body over from the hips. Keep your back flat and hips square. Place your left hand on your right shin or, for advanced students, on the floor outside the right foot.

● Press with your left hand into the floor or leg, while raising your right arm upward, with fingertips pointing to the sky. Turn your head and chest to look along the right arm; focus on the hand. Hold for five breaths.

● Release the position, raising your left arm out to the side. Slowly turn your body to the front as you return to the upright position.

● Turn your feet so that they are parallel to each other, and hold your outstretched arms at shoulder height. Turn your head to face forward and repeat on the left side.

exhale   ‖   **inhale**   ▶   ‖

extended side angle *utthita parsvakonasana*

Good alignment of the chest, hips, and legs will help you hold this position. Use your fingertips to touch the floor if it is too difficult to place the hand flat.

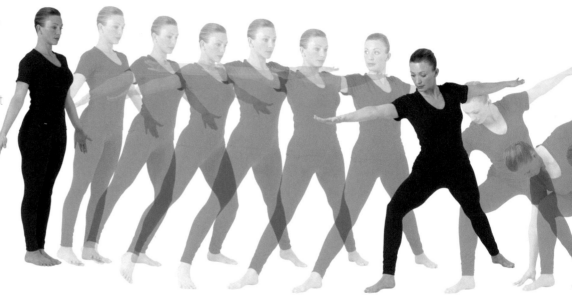

● Start in the standing position; step the feet apart by one and a half leg's length. Extend the arms out to shoulder height. Engage the thigh muscles and relax the shoulders.

● Turn the right foot out to the side by 90 degrees, and turn the left foot inward by 10 to 15 degrees. Turn your head to the right.

● Engage the thighs and press both feet firmly into the floor to create a stable base for the extended stretch.

▶ inhale   ▶ exhale   ▶ inhale   ▶

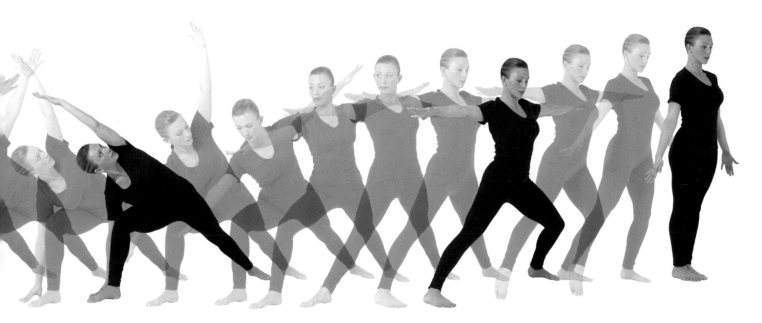

● Bend your right leg so that your shin is vertical and your thigh parallel to the floor. Keep your knee in line with but not beyond the ankle. Lower your right hand and place it on the floor, outside the right foot.

● Raise your left arm into the air and take it over to the left side of your head. Turn your chin to the left shoulder and focus on your left hand. Keep your left leg outstretched and both feet firmly on the floor.

● Hold this position for five breaths, making sure that your hips, chest, and legs are kept in line with each other.

● Lift your body into the upright position, raising your arms to shoulder height and straighten your leg. Turn your head to the front and keep your feet parallel, then repeat the sequence to the left.

exhale   **inhale**   ▶   ▶   **II**

revolving side angle *parivrtta parsvakonasana*

This movement is the twisted version of the Extended Side Angle. It gives a strong twist to the spine, helping to rejuvenate the spinal column.

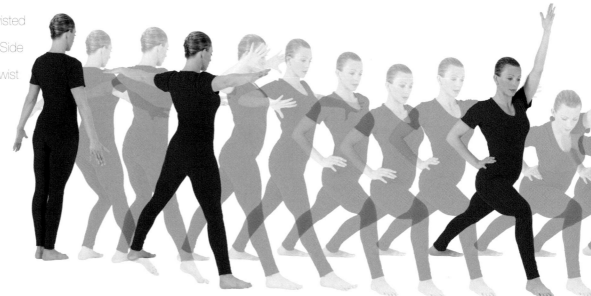

● Start in the standing position; step the feet apart by one and a half leg's length. Extend the arms out to shoulder height. Engage the thigh muscles and relax the shoulders.

● Turn your right foot to the side by 90 degrees, and your left foot toward the body by 45 degrees. Turn to face the right leg with hips square. Bend your right leg so the shin is vertical and the thigh parallel to the floor.

● Put your right hand on your hip. Raise your left arm overhead, with fingertips pointing to the sky.

▶ inhale   exhale   ▶ inhale   ▶

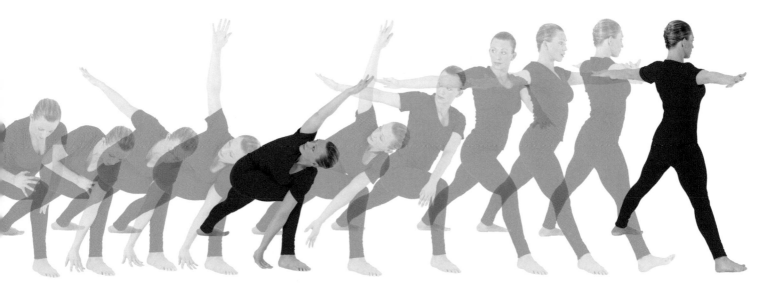

● Folding the body over, take the left elbow to the outside of your right knee and press the palms together. Beginners should hold this position for five breaths.

● For advanced people, put your left hand on the floor outside your right foot, raising the right arm overhead. Look along your right arm. Tuck in your chin, keep your neck in line with your spine and focus on the hand.

● Release this position after five breaths by lifting your left hand off the floor. Slowly take your left arm to the side and lower the right arm. Hold them at shoulder height.

● Lift your body upright and turn it to the front. Turn your head forward and your feet parallel. Repeat the sequence to the left.

exhale ▶ inhale ▶ ‖

forward bend "a" *prasarita padottanasana "a"*

This is the first of four versions of the Forward Bend movement. As a beginner, you may find the position difficult to hold but, with practice, your flexibility will improve greatly.

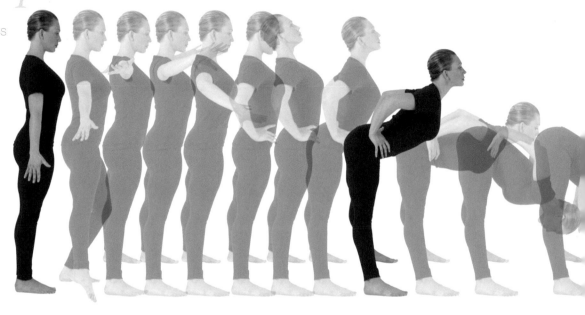

● Start in the standing pose with feet together and arms by your sides. Step your feet apart to one and half leg's length and make sure they are parallel. Raise your outstretched arms to shoulder height.

● Place your hands on your hips. Lift the chest and look up, making sure not to arch the lower back.

● Fold forward from the hips, taking the chest toward the knees. Keep your back straight. Release your hands from the hips and place them on the floor between the feet.

▶ **exhale**   **inhale**   ▶   **exhale**   ▶

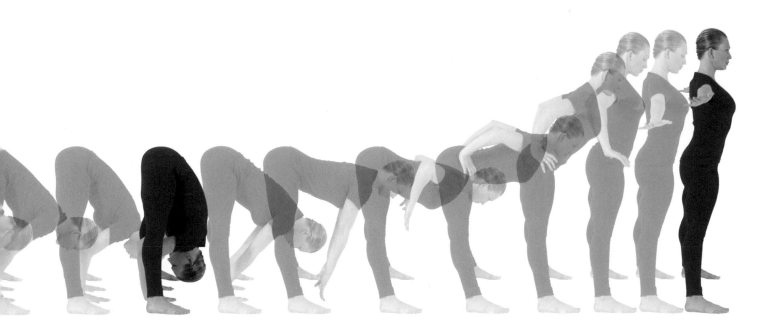

● Press your palms against the floor, keeping your arms straight, and focus on a point between your legs. Keep your chest away from the hips. Hold this position for five breaths.

● Raise your hands onto their fingertips, and slowly lift the chest away from your legs. Lift your head to look forward.

● Place your hands on your hips and keep your chest open. Lift your body to upright.

● Raise your arms out to the side and lift your head upright.

exhale ▶ inhale   exhale   inhale ▶   II

forward bend "b"

prasarita padottanasana "b"

The aim of this variation of the
Forward Bend is to intensify
the leg stretch and develop
your leg muscles. It also
increases the flex in your hips.

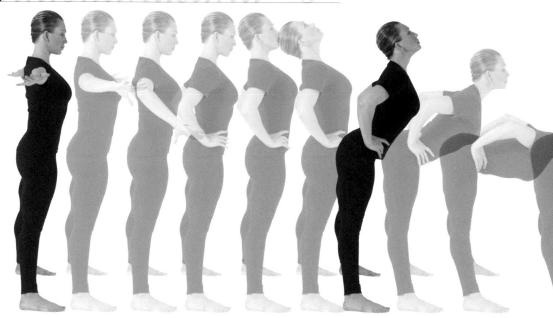

● Place your hands on your hips,
open your chest and roll your
shoulders back.

● Lift the chest and look up, making
sure not to arch the lower back.

● Fold forward from the hips. Keep
your back straight and make sure that
your neck is in line with your spine.

▶ **exhale**　　　　**inhale**　　　　▶　　**exhale**　　　　▶

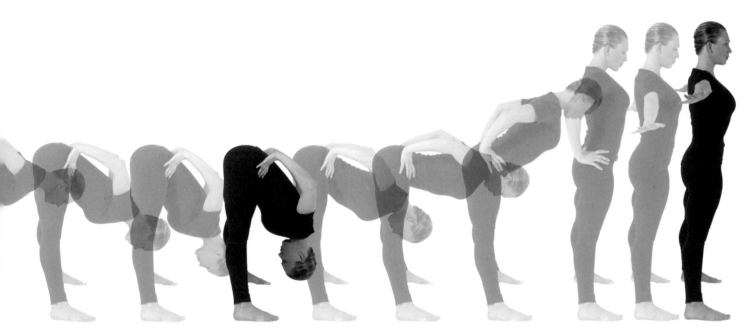

● Your body should be fully folded, with the crown of your head pointing toward the floor. Keep your chest away from the hips and tuck your chin in. Hold this position for five breaths.

● Release the position, slowly lifting the chest away from your legs. Keep your hands on your hips.

● Continue lifting the body to an upright position, keeping your legs apart as you straighten from the hips.

● Extend the arms to shoulder height, keeping the shoulders relaxed and away from your ears.

exhale   ‖   ▶   inhale   inhale   ‖

forward bend "c"

prasarita padottanasana "c"

This Forward Bend combines the hip fold with an arm and shoulder stretch. Remember to keep the breathing soft and regular when you hold the Forward Bend position.

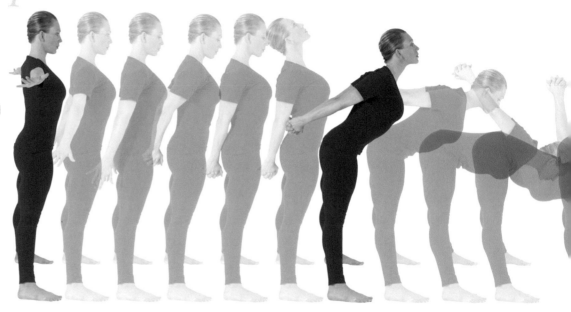

● Interlock your hands behind your back and squeeze your shoulder blades together

● Inhale as you roll your shoulders back, lift your chest, and look up.

● Bending forward from the hips, fold your body toward your legs. Keep your back straight and your neck in line with your spine. With hands still clasped, raise your outstretched arms behind your back as you fold over.

▶ **exhale**   **inhale**   ▶ **exhale**   ▶

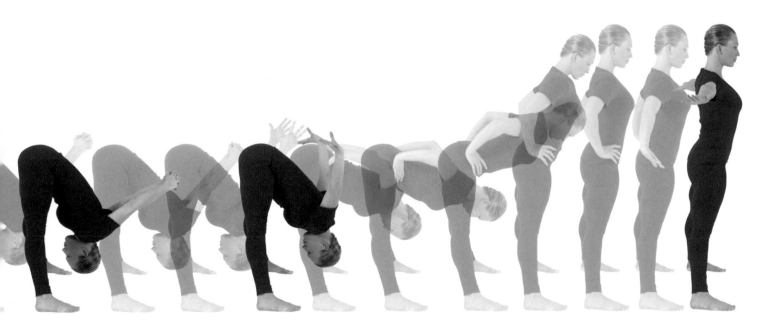

● With the crown of your head pointing at the floor take your arms over your head towards the floor. Keep your chest away from the hips and tuck your chin in. Hold this position for five breaths.

● Release the position, slowly lifting the chest away from your legs. Tilt your head back slightly to keep it in line with the neck. Unclasp your hands and place them on your hips.

● Unfold the body from the hips, but keep your hands on your hips for support.

● When the torso is upright, extend the arms out to shoulder height.

inhale   exhale   ▶   inhale   ▶   exhale   II

forward bend "d"

prasarita padottanasana "d"

This final version of the Forward Bend can be combined with the Hands to Toes and Feet movements shown on pages 36–39. Until you become well-practiced in this Forward Bend, you may find it more comfortable to hold your ankles rather than your toes.

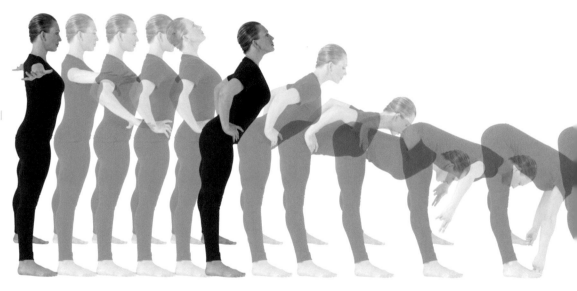

● Place your hands on your hips and open your chest.

● Inhale, then roll the shoulders back, lift the chest, and look up.

● Fold forward from the hips. Lift your hands from your hips and lower them to your feet. Depending on your reach, hook your big toe with your forefinger or grasp hold of your ankles.

▶ **exhale**   **inhale** ▶   **exhale**   ▶

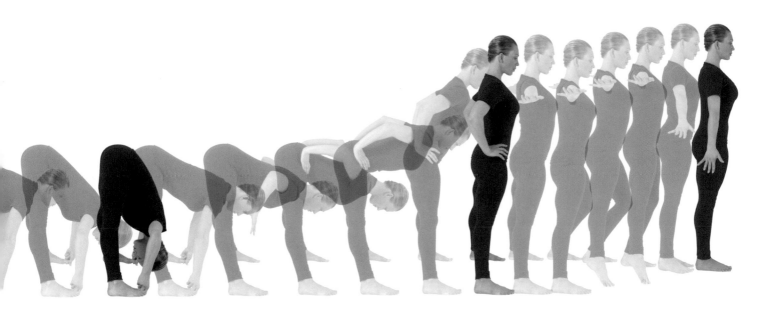

● Lift your chest, and hold your head up to look forward. Keep your chest away from your hips and move your shoulders from your ears. Exhale: fold forward, move your chest to your knees, and bend your elbows.

● Release this position after five breaths, slowly lifting the chest away from your legs. Unhook the big toes and place your hands on the hips. Tilt your head back slightly to keep it in line with the neck.

● Continue lifting the body from the hips, and keep your hands on your hips for support.

● In the standing position, lift your arms out to the sides and step your feet together, with toes pointing forward. Slowly lower your arms to the sides and breathe deeply.

inhale   exhale   inhale   inhale   ▶   ‖

intense side stretch

parsvottanasana

When practiced regularly, this movement improves the flexibility in your hips and helps to relieve any stiffness in your legs and hips. Reverse *Namaste*, the Prayer pose, is formed by pressing the palms of your hands together behind the back.

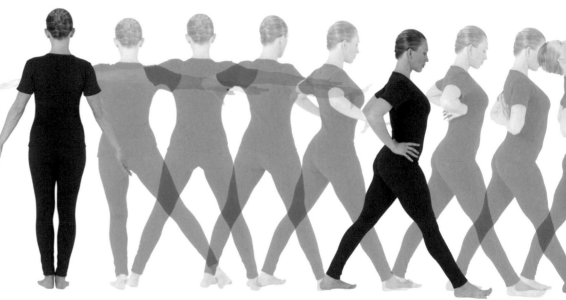

● Start in the standing position with feet together and arms by your sides. Step your feet apart to one leg's length. Raise your outstretched arms to shoulder height.

● Turn your right foot out to the side by 90 degrees, and turn your left foot toward the body by 40 degrees. Place your hands on your hips, and turn your head and hips to face the right leg.

● Take your hands behind your back, pressing the palms together in Reverse *Namaste*. If this is not comfortable, clasp your elbows instead. Lift your chest and and your head to look toward the sky.

▶ **inhale**　　　　**exhale**　　▶　　**inhale**　　　▶

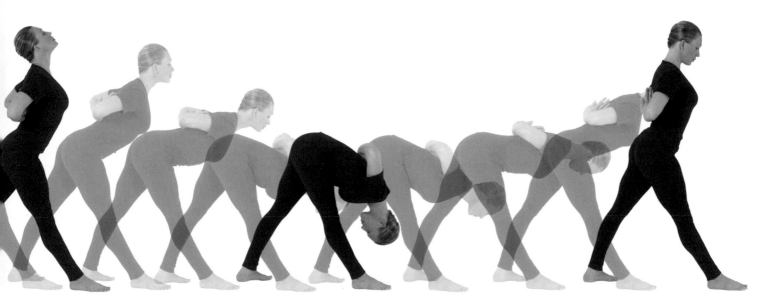

● Fold your body over your right leg, keeping your hips square. Take your chest toward your knees and tuck your chin in, so that the crown of your head is pointing toward the floor. Hold this position for five breaths.

● Release the position, slowly lifting your chest away from the knees. Keep the head and neck in line with the spine as you unfold.

● Continue lifting the body from the hips to an upright position.

● Keeping the hands in the same position, turn to face the left leg. Now repeat on the left side.

exhale ❙❙ ▶ **inhale** ▶ **exhale** ❙❙

extended leg *uttbita basta padangusthasana*

The balance required to
perform this movement well
will strengthen your leg
muscles and improve your
steadiness and poise.
Beginners may prefer to
keep the leg bent.

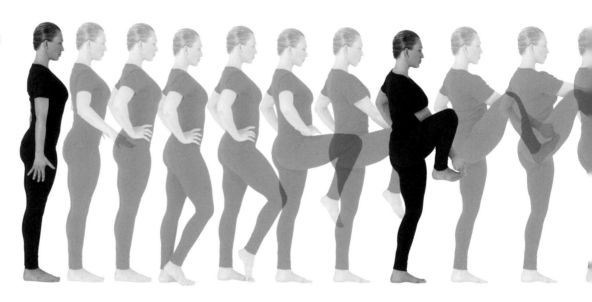

● Start in the standing position, with
feet together and arms by your sides.
Place your hands on the hips.

● Lift your right foot off the floor and
bend your leg. Slowly raise your right
knee in front of you, and hook the
big toe of your right foot with your
thumb and forefinger. Keep the left leg
straight but without locking the knee.

● Extend your right leg, still holding
onto your right foot. Keep your left
hand on your hip. Relax the shoulders,
making sure they are level; keep your
hips and shoulders square and your
chest open. Hold for five breaths.

▶ **inhale**
▶ **exhale**

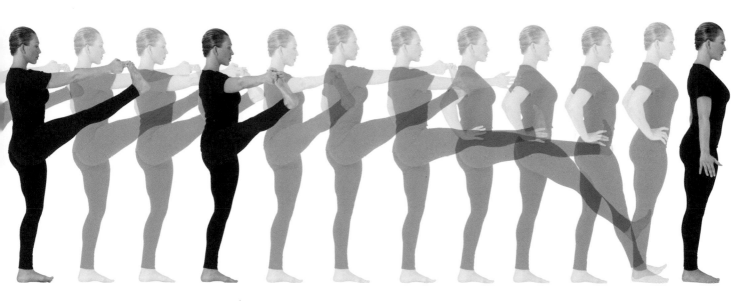

● Lift and open the chest and take the raised leg out to the right. Keeping your hips and shoulders square, turn your head to look over your left shoulder. Hold the pose for five breaths and exhale.

● Bring the leg back to the front and look forward again, keeping the chest open and the thigh engaged.

● Release the toe, bringing the hand back to the hip, and hold the leg up. Hold this pose for five breaths.

● Slowly lower the leg and return to the standing position. Pause a moment before repeating the sequence with the left leg and arm.

inhale   exhale   ‖   inhale   ▶   exhale   ‖

the tree *vrksasana*

This movement concentrates on improving your balance and poise. Use your breathing to help you focus and center your balance.

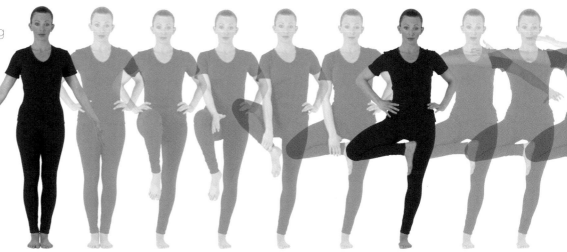

● Start in the standing position with feet together and arms by your sides. Raise your arms to place your hands on your hips.

● Lift your right foot off the floor and bend your right leg, bringing the knee to the front. Take hold of your right ankle in your right hand, and guide the sole of the foot into the inside of your left leg.

● Take the foot as high as possible and press it firmly against the leg. Place your right hand on the hip again.

▶ **inhale**　　　　　▶ **exhale**　　　　▶

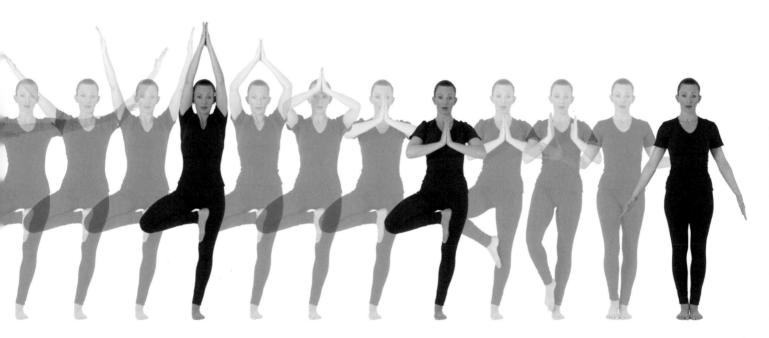

● Slowly raise your arms over your head, pressing the palms together. Focus on a point in front of you; keep the standing leg strong and straight.

● Hold this position for five breaths; then slowly lower the arms in front of you, keeping the palms together.

● When the hands reach chest height, start to slide your right foot down the side of the left leg, and take it to the ground.

● Release your palms from the Prayer position and take your arms out to the sides. Bring both feet together, with toes pointing forward in the standing position.

inhale   ‖   ▶   exhale   ‖

fierce posture

uthatasana

To appreciate this movement, imagine that you are sitting in an chair and then getting up from it without the support of the chair arms. This sequence is very good for toning the thighs and buttocks.

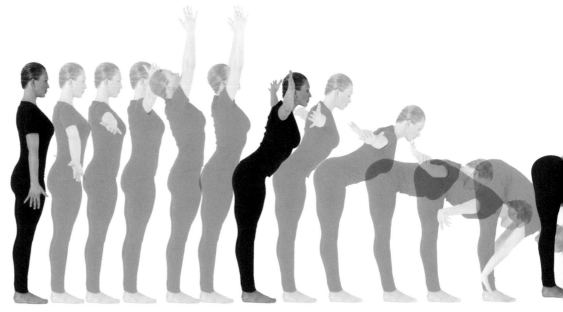

● Start by standing with your feet together and toe joints and ankles touching. Engage the thighs and pull your stomach in and upwards. Relax your shoulder. Extend your arms down and out from the shoulders.

● Rotate your arms out to the sides, turning the palms so that they face outward. Take the arms up above your head, pressing the palms together, and then look up at your hands.

● Fold forward from the hips, as you bring your arms out and down to the sides. Keeping your torso lengthened, take your chest toward your knees so your ribs move away from your hips.

▶   **inhale**   ▶   **exhale**   ▶

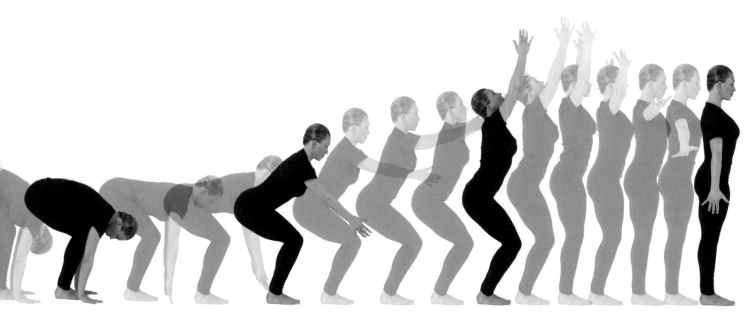

● Bend your knees and drop your bottom toward the heels, keeping the heels of the feet firmly pressing into the floor.

● Lift the torso away from the bent legs, bringing the arms up with the palms pressing together.

● Look up and hold the position for five breaths.

● Return to the standing position by straightening the legs, taking the arms to your side, and looking forward.

inhale ▶ ‖ exhale ▶ ‖

warrior "a"

virabhadrasana "a"

This is the first of two versions of the Warrior movement. Remember always to keep the bent knee in line with, and not beyond, the ankle when holding this position.

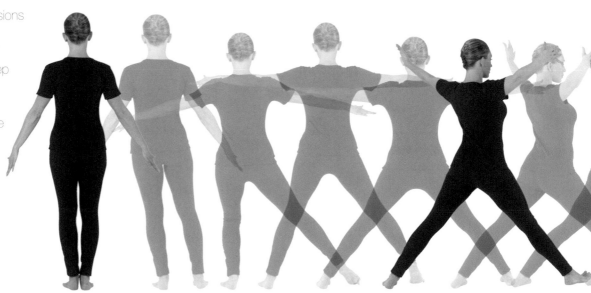

● Start in the standing position, with feet together and arms by your sides. Engage the thighs and pull your stomach in. Relax your shoulders.

● Step your feet apart to one and half leg's length and make sure they are parallel. Raise your outstretched arms to shoulder height.

● Turn your right foot out to the side by 90 degrees. Turn your left foot inward to an angle of 45 degrees. Take your arms overhead and press the palms together. Tilt back your head to focus on the hands.

▶ **inhale**   **exhale**   ▶   **inhale**   ▶

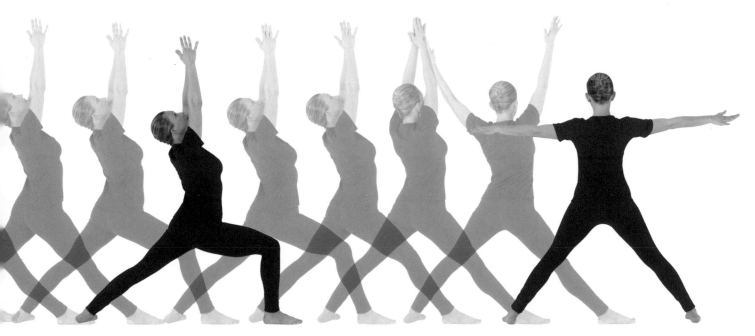

● Bend your right leg so that the shin is vertical and the thigh is parallel to the floor. Keep your left leg straight, and press the whole of the left foot firmly on the floor. Don't collapse your lower back; hold for five breaths.

● Slowly turn the body toward the front, at the same time releasing your hands. Lower the arms to shoulder height, keeping them outstretched.

● Turn your feet to the front, with toes pointing forward. Keep your back straight and the head upright.

● Repeat the movement on the left side.

exhale ❚❚   inhale ▶   exhale   ▶   ❚❚

warrior "b"

To obtain as full a stretch as possible when holding the Warrior position, imagine that your arms are being pulled in opposite directions to each other.

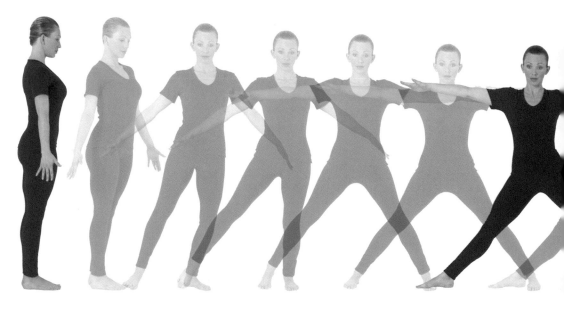

● Start in the standing position with feet together and arms by your sides. Engage the thighs and focus on the Bhandas. Try to keep your shoulders relaxed.

● Step your feet apart to one and half leg's length and make sure they are parallel. Raise your outstretched arms to shoulder height.

● Turn your right foot out to the side by 90 degrees. Turn your left foot inward to an angle of 10–15 degrees. Turn your head to the right to focus on the hands.

inhale ▶ **exhale** ▶ **inhale** ▶

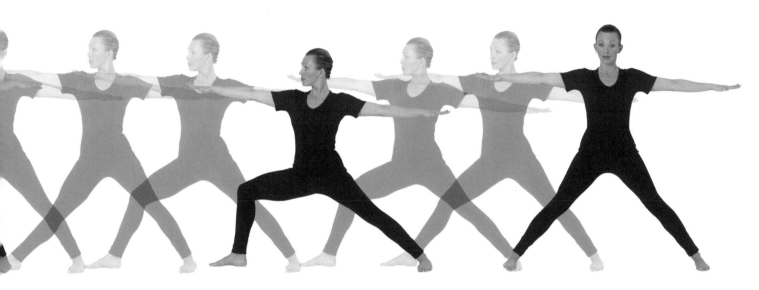

● Bend your right leg so that the shin is vertical and the thigh is parallel to the floor.

● Keep your left leg straight, and press the whole of the left foot firmly on the floor. Hold this position for five breaths and exhale.

● Slowly straighten the right leg as you bring the feet back to parallel; and look forward.

● Repeat the movement on the left side.

exhale ❚❚ ▶ **inhale** ▶ ❚❚

half vinyasa

from upright to seated

The half *Vinyasa* takes you from the standing position, through Downward Dog, and into the seated position. As you work through this sequence, keep your movements smooth and harmonious.

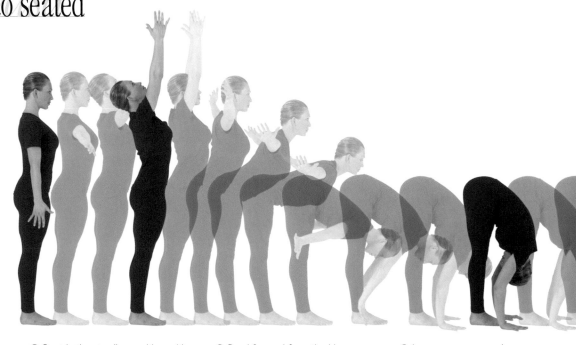

● Start in the standing position, with feet together and arms by your sides. Take the arms up above your head, pressing the palms together. Look up.

● Bend forward from the hips, Keeping your torso lengthened, take your chest toward your knees so that your ribs move away from your hips.

● Lower your arms and press your palms against the floor, either side of your feet. Tuck your chin into the chest and point the crown of your head toward the ground.

▶ inhale   exhale   ▶   ▶

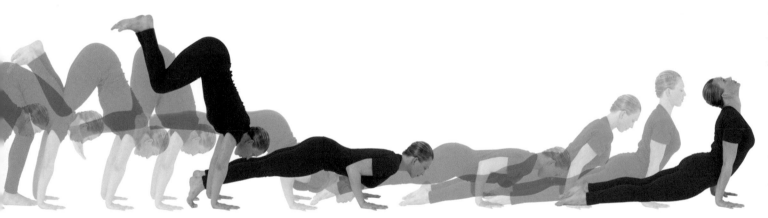

● Pushing into your hands, lift the chest and extend your torso and look up and out.

● With your hands flat and bending your knees if necessary, transfer your body weight from the feet to the hands. Lift your hips high and jump back, landing with the toes curled under and the elbows tucked in.

● Roll your feet over your toes and take the chest forward. Make sure the body is parallel to the floor.

● Straighten your arms, lift up the chest, and tilt the head upward. Press the feet into the floor so the knees come off the floor. This is the Upward Dog position. This sequence continues on the next page.

inhale   exhale   ▶ inhale   ▶

from upright to seated

The half *Vinyasa* is used throughout the seated postures to divide each of the sequences.

Its purpose is to get the blood flowing through the body after each seated *asana*. Look for the

indicators in the captions to find out when to insert the half *Vinyasa* in your routine.

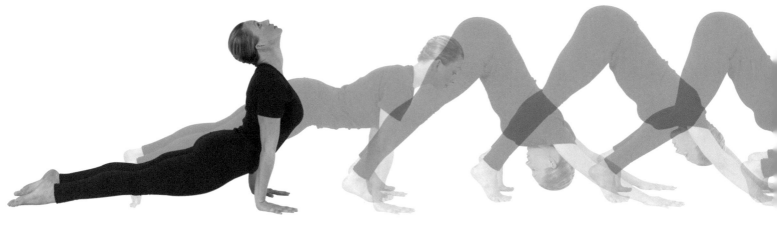

● Your spine, thighs, and legs should be fully extended. Keep your chest open and lift your chin.

● Release the pose and and gently bring your head upright, with eyes looking downward. Keep your arms straight.

● Roll your feet back over the toes, lifting your bottom high into the air.

● Push against the floor with the palms of your hands. Aim to press your heels into the floor and point your buttocks upward to create an inverted "V"-shape. Hold this position for the inhale breath.

▶ **inhale**   **exhale**   ▶   **inhale**   ▶

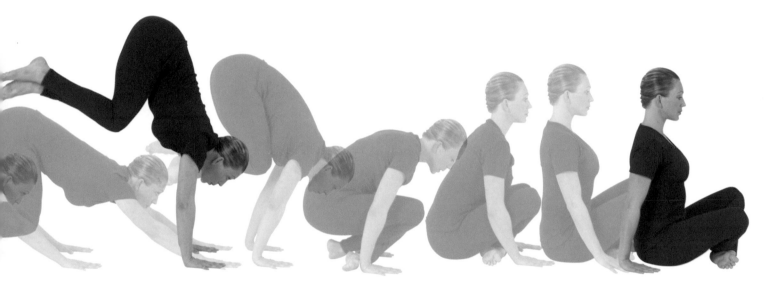

● Bend your knees and focus your eyes on a point beyond your hands.

● Push your feet away from the ground, carrying your hips high as you jump.

● Cross your legs in mid air; then bring your feet to land inside the outstretched arms.

● Tuck your buttocks under your body. Place your crossed legs in front of you, and slide your palms backward to support the pose.

exhale   ‖   **inhale**   ▶   ▶   ▶   ‖

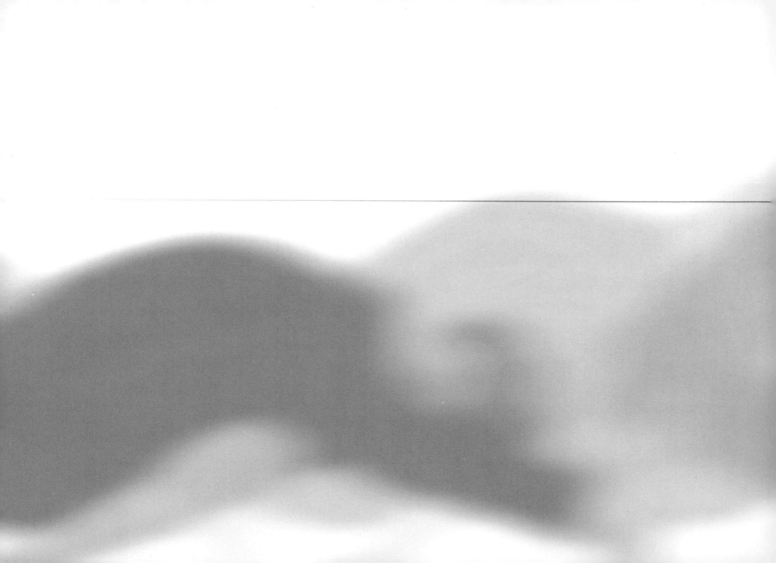

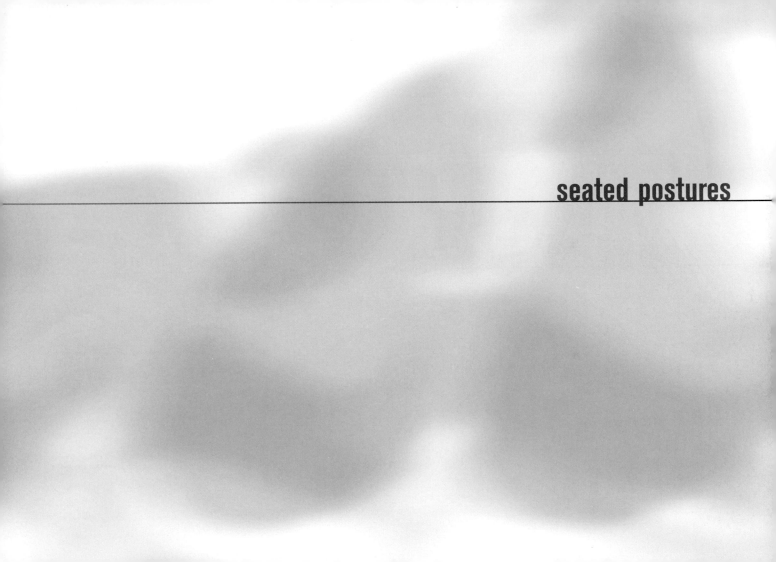

seated postures

the rod to forward bend *paschimottasana*

This sequence includes the Rod position and the Forward Bend, both of which allow you to extend and soften the spine fully. They are highly valued positions because they ease the spinal compression caused by standing upright.

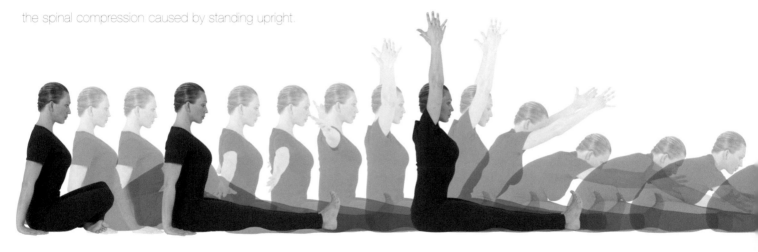

● Start in the seated position with crossed legs in front of you and palms pressed against the floor, positioned by your bottom, at shoulder's width. Keep your back and neck straight, and push your chest forward.

● Uncross your legs and extend them in front of you so that ankle joints and big toes are touching. Press the hands into the floor by the hips to help keep the spine straight. Hold this position (the Rod) for five breaths.

● Looking straight ahead, lift your hands off the floor and extend your arms out to the sides. Take them above your head, palms facing inward.

● Slowly fold the body forward, moving your chest toward the knees. Keep your spine as straight as possible. Grasp the outside edges of your feet with both hands. Tuck your chin in and hold for five breaths.

▶　　　❚❚　　inhale　　　▶　　　　　　▶　　exhale　　　▶

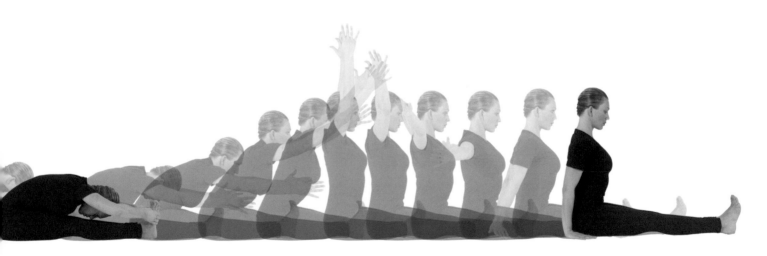

● If this position does not feel comfortable, slide your hands down to your ankles and take hold of them.

● Extend your arms out by your ears as you lift the torso away from the legs to an upright position.

● Slowly lower the arms down to your sides and position them either side of your bottom, with palms pressed against the floor.

● Keep your back and neck straight and hold your head upright. Now perform the half *Vinyasa* before going on to the next *asana*.

❚❚   ▶   **inhale**   **exhale**   ▶   ❚❚

counterpose to forward bend

This movement starts in the *Dandasana*, or Rod position, and takes you through the counterpose to the Forward Bend. It provides an intense stretch across the front of the body.

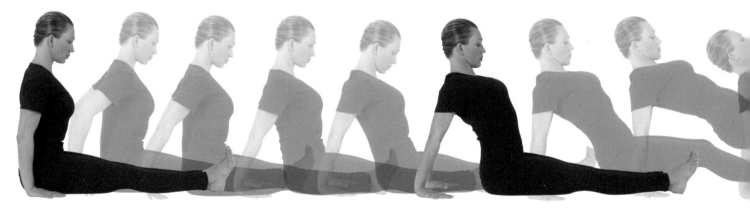

● Sit on the floor with your legs stretched in front. Your ankle and toe joints should be touching and the toes pointing upward. Place your hands on the floor about six inches behind you, shoulder width apart.

● Press your hands into the floor as you lift your chest. Keep your eyes focused on your toes.

● Bend your knees slightly so that the soles of your feet move toward the floor. Keep your chest lifted.

● Press the soles of your feet firmly into the floor, as you push your hips forward and up toward the sky.

inhale ▶ **exhale** ▶ **inhale** ▶

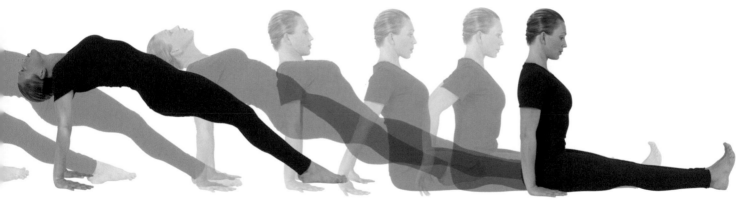

● Relax your head back—do not force it back. Hold this position for five breaths.

● Slowly lower your bottom toward the floor. Bring the head and chest upright and look forward.

● Bring your arms forward to the starting position and let your gaze lower to your toes.

● With legs fully extended, point your toes upward, keeping your heels firmly on the floor.

exhale ‖ ▶ exhale inhale ▶ ‖

jump from the rod

This sequence includes three asanas, namely the Crocodile and Upward and Downward Dog.

Until you have become well-practiced in the movement, you might find it easier to step the legs

backward or forward rather than jump forward and back.

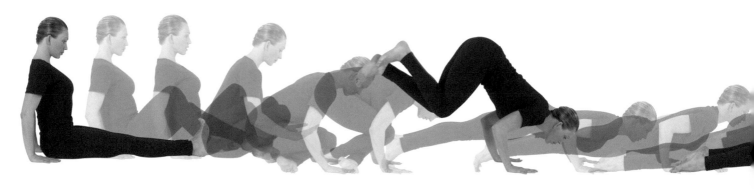

● Sit on the floor with your legs outstretched in front. The ankle and toe joints should be touching and your the toes pointing upward. Place your hands on the floor, on either side of your hips, fingertips facing forward.

● Bring your knees toward the chest and cross your legs in the process. Take your arms around the outside of your knees as you place your hands on the floor in front of you.

● Roll over the feet onto your hands and knees. With your hands flat, lift your hips, and jump your legs back.

● Land with your toes curled under, your elbows tucked in, and the body parallel to the floor.

▶ **inhale**   **exhale**   ▶   ▶

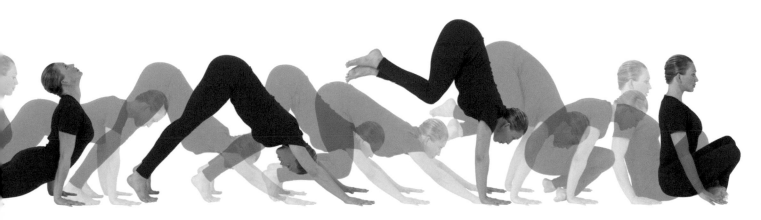

● Roll your feet over your toes, taking the chest forward at the same time. Straighten your arms, lift up the chest, and tilt the head upward. Press the feet into the floor so the knees lift. This is Upward Dog.

● Bring your head upright, with eyes looking down. Keep your arms straight. Roll your feet back over the toes, lift your bottom high, and into Downward Dog. Hold for the inhale breath.

● Press your hands and your feet into the floor. Bend your knees and look at your hands. On an inhale, push your feet away from the floor, carrying the hips high as you jump forward.

● Cross your legs in midair; then bring your feet to land inside the extended arms. Tuck your bottom under your body. Place your crossed legs in front of you and place your palms on the floor.

inhale   exhale   ▶   inhale   exhale   inhale   ▶   II

forward bend to the knees

Keep the thigh of the outstretched leg engaged to stop it rolling out. If you cannot catch your foot in this sequence, use the ankle instead. Be sure not to force the movement.

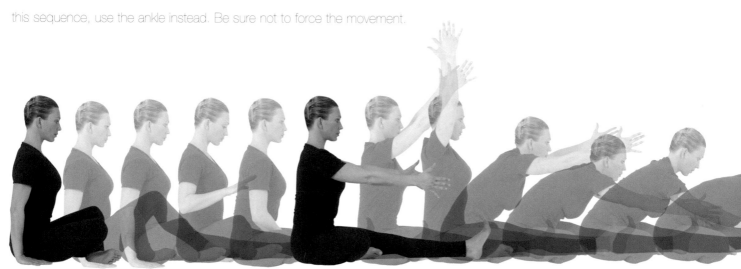

● Sit on the floor with your legs crossed in front of you and the soles of your feet facing out to the sides. Place your hands by your thighs, with palms pressed on the floor, and fingertips pointing forward.

● Slowly extend your left leg out in front of you. Keeping your right leg bent, press the sole of your right foot against the inside of your left thigh. Keep your neck and back straight.

● Extend both arms in front of you, and raise them overhead, with fingertips pointing upward.

● Slowly fold the body forward from the hips, taking your chest down toward your knees.

▶   **exhale**   **inhale**   ▶   **exhale**   ▶

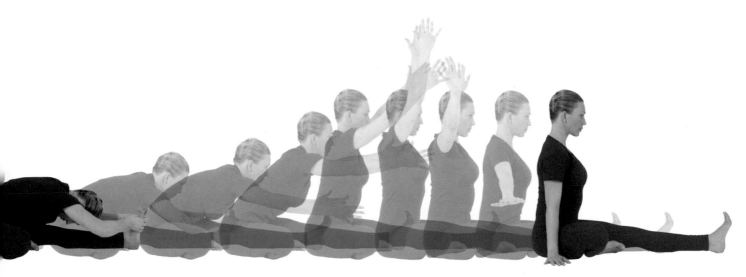

● Take hold of your left foot with both hands. Tuck your chin into your chest and keep your shoulders square as you move them away from your ears. Hold for five breaths.

● Release the foot and slowly lift your chest away from your knees. Keep your back extended and hold your arms in front of you.

● Continue lifting the chest upward, keeping your head upright. Take your arms above your head; then lower them to your sides. Keep the left leg extended, heel resting on the floor, and the right leg tucked into the thigh.

● Place your hands on the floor by your sides. Relax and breathe in; then repeat the movement on the right side. Pause and then perform the half *Vinyasa* before the next *asana*.

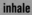 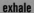

marichi position "a"

marichyasana "a"

This movement is dedicated to Marichi, who was the grandfather of the Sun god. If you find it uncomfortable to clasp your wrist behind your back, catch hold of your palms or fingers instead. If this is still difficult, hold a belt between your hands.

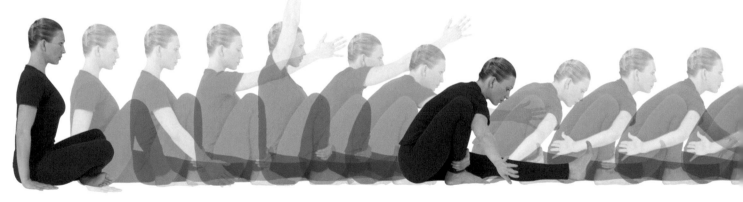

● Sit on the floor with your legs crossed in front of you and the soles of your feet facing out to the sides. Place your hands by your thighs, with palms pressed on the floor, and fingertips pointing forward.

● Slowly extend your left leg to the front. Bend your right leg and place the sole of your foot parallel to, but not touching, the inside thigh of the left leg. With your left hand, grasp your right shin and hold it vertical.

● Extend your right arm and raise it overhead, with the fingertips pointing upward. Focus your eyes in front. Slowly fold the body forward to the inside of the right leg. Release the right shin, taking your left arm behind you.

● Wrap your right arm around the front of your right shin, and take it behind your back to catch hold of your left wrist.

inhale ▶ exhale ▶ ▶

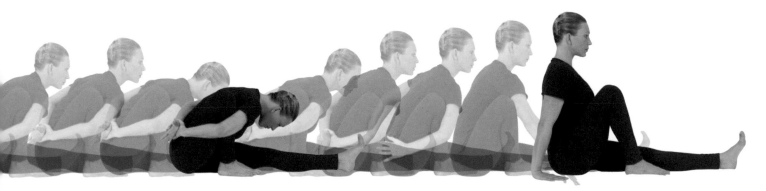

● Continue lowering your chest toward your knees. Keep your neck and spine aligned throughout and your shoulders parallel to the floor. Make sure that the back of your extended left leg stays on the floor.

● Take your body as low as is comfortable. Tuck your chin into your chest and gaze downward. Hold the position for five breaths.

● Release your arms and slowly bring them to the front of the body. Raise your chest upward, keeping your neck and spine straight. Place your right foot parallel to your left knee.

● Place your hands by the sides of your bottom, with palms facing forward. Repeat on the right side. Now perform the half *Vinyasa* before starting the next *asana*.

▶   **inhale**   ‖ **exhale** ▶   ‖

marichi position "c"

Both versions of this movement concentrate on the thoracic region of the spine, and
improve the blood circulation in your body. Once again, if you cannot hold your hands
behind your back, use a belt adjusted to the limit of your flexibility.

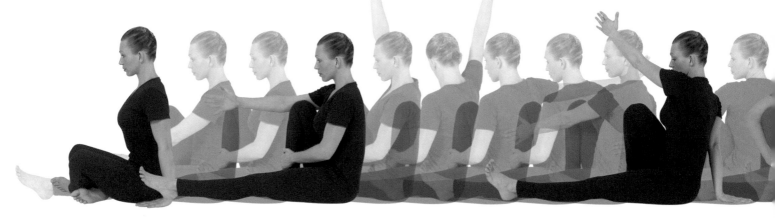

● Sit on the floor with your legs
crossed in front of you, and the soles
of your feet facing out to the sides.
Place your hands by your thighs, with
palms pressed on the floor and
fingertips pointing forward.

● Slowly extend your left leg to the
front. Bend your right leg and place
the sole of your foot parallel to, but
not touching, the inside thigh of the
left leg. With your left hand, grasp your
right shin and hold it vertical.

● Extend your right arm and raise it
overhead, with the fingertips pointing
upward. Focus your eyes in front.
Keeping your hips square, slowly turn
the body from the thoracic spine to
look over your right shoulder.

● Lower your right arm and take
it behind your back, placing your
palm on the floor with fingertips
pointing away from you.

exhale ▶ inhale ▶ exhale ▶

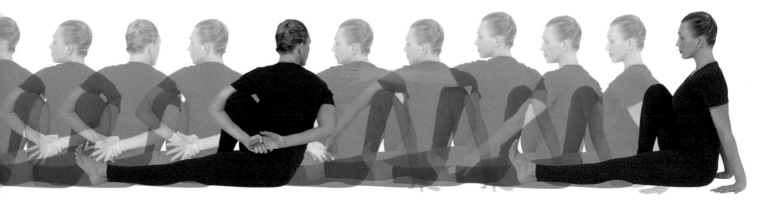

● Release the right shin, taking your left arm around the front of the shin. On the exhale, wrap the left arm behind you to grasp the right wrist, palm or fingers.

● Make sure that the back of your extended left leg stays in contact with the floor. Hold for five breaths.

● Release the hands and let your upper body uncoil to face the front. Bring your arms beside you.

● Straighten your neck and spine, and hold your head upright with hands on the floor behind you. Now repeat on the left side. Now perform the half *Vinyasa* before you start the next *asana*.

inhale   exhale   inhale   ▶   exhale   II

the boat *sana*

This movement focuses on improving your balance and strengthening your legs and stomach. If you find it uncomfortable to hold your legs up at angle of 45 degrees, bend your legs at the knees and keep your shins parallel to the floor.

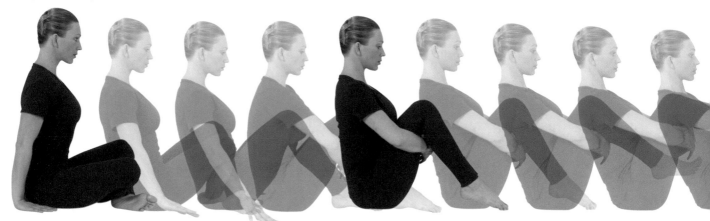

● Sit on the floor with your legs crossed in front of you and the soles of your feet facing out to the sides. Place your hands by your thighs, with palms pressed on the floor and fingertips pointing forward.

● Slowly uncross your legs and wrap your arms underneath your thighs. Clasp your hands together at the backs of your knees.

● Take your shoulders away from your ears and straighten your spine. Lift your chest as you raise your feet off the floor, and bring your knees in toward your body.

● Slowly extend your legs to an angle of 45 degrees. Keep your spine straight and your chest lifted, and relax your shoulders. Focus your eyes on your toes.

exhale ▶ **inhale** ▶ **exhale** ▶

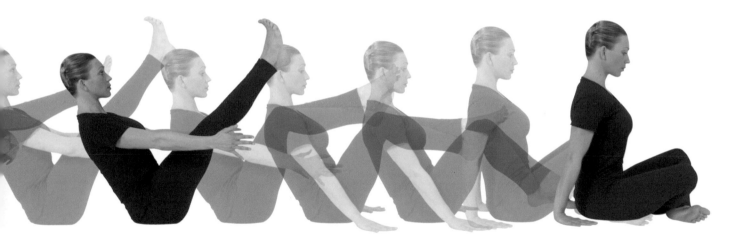

● Release your hands, keeping your arms parallel to the floor as you reach out in front of you. Hold this position for five breaths.

● Release the position, lowering your arms to the ground. Press your palms on the floor, with the fingertips pointing forward. Slowly lower your legs toward the ground, keeping the movement as smooth as possible.

● As your feet touch the ground, bring your body into the upright seated position. Slide your hands behind you and position them either side of your bottom for support.

● Cross your legs as you bring them in toward your body. Keep your spine and neck straight and look forward.

inhale   **exhale** ▶   **inhale** ▶

feet around hands *half vinyasa*

This movement takes you from the seated position, through the Crocodile and Downward and Upward Dog positions. In the final jump, your feet land around the outside of your hands. Until you feel confident enough to jump, you may step your feet backward or forward.

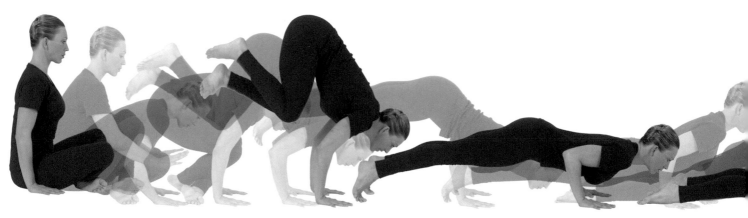

● Sit on the floor with your legs crossed together and the soles facing out to the sides. Place your hands on the floor either side of your bottom, and point your fingertips forward.

● Slide your hands out in front of you and shift your body weight onto your palms. With feet still crossed, raise your heels off the ground. Bend your knees and focus on a point beyond your hands.

● Push your feet away from the ground, carrying your hips high as you jump back. Uncross your legs in the air.

● Land with your toes curled under your feet, the elbows tucked in, and the body parallel to the floor.

inhale ▶ exhale ▶ ▶

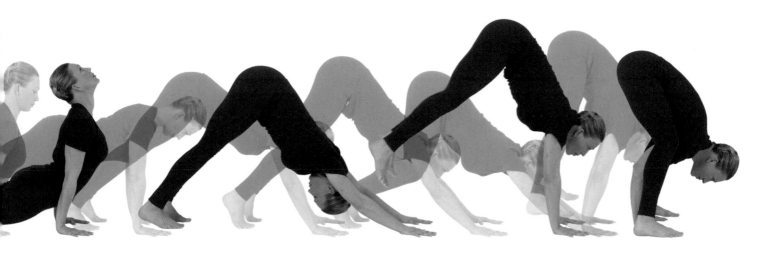

● Roll your feet over your toes, taking the chest forward at the same time. Straighten your arms, lift up the chest, and tilt the head upward. Press the feet into the floor so the knees lift off. This is Upward Dog.

● Bring your head upright, with eyes looking down. Keep your arms straight. Roll your feet back over the toes, lift your bottom high and into Downward Dog. Hold for the inhale breath.

● Bend your knees and focus on a point beyond your hands. On the inhale breath, push your feet away from the ground, carrying your hips high as you jump.

● Bring your feet to land outside of your hands, keeping your legs slightly bent. This sequence continues on the next page.

inhale   exhale   ▶   inhale   exhale   inhale   ▶   ▶

feet around arms *bhujapidasana*

The arms, wrists, and hands derive benefits from this movement, although you will find that it also strengthens the abdominal muscles. Every part of your body is used as a weight or counterweight in this movement, while your hands and arms provide the pivot.

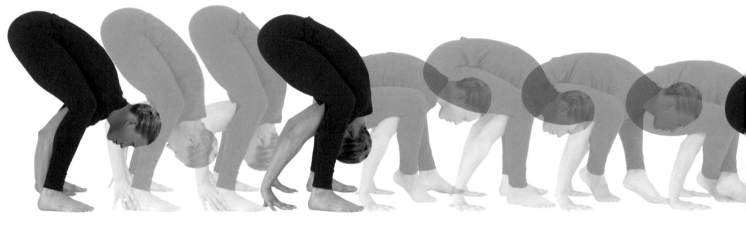

● Continue from the last page, looking straight down at the floor with hands between your feet.

● Lift your hands and place them on the floor behind your heels. Gently ease your shoulders to the backs of your knees; then start to walk your feet toward each other.

● Slide your hands further behind your feet, and tuck your chin into your chest. Squeeze your upper arms with your thighs and, as your feet come together, cross them at the ankles. Press your hands into the floor.

● Slowly transfer your body weight onto your hands. Still squeezing with the thighs, lift your bottom up and raise your feet off the ground and away from you. Hold for five breaths.

▶ **inhale**   **exhale**   ▶ **inhale**   ▶ **exhale**   ▶

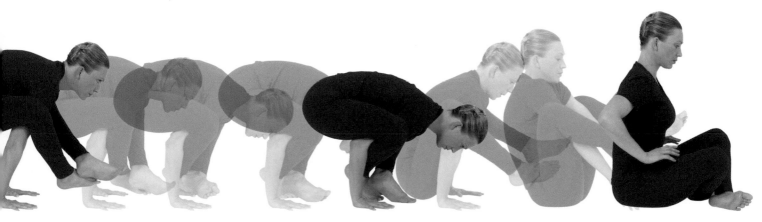

● Release the position slowly, lowering your feet to the ground and placing them in between your hands.

● Tilt forward slightly to balance; then lower your bottom to bring your body into an upright position.

● As your bottom touches the ground, uncross your feet and place them on the floor.

● Lift your hands off the floor and bring them to rest on the tops of your thighs. Keeping your legs bent, cross them over with soles facing out to the sides. Now perform the half *Vinyasa*.

inhale   ▶   exhale   inhale   ▶   11

the turtle *asana*

The Turtle *asana* increases the flex in the hips, stretches the lower spine, and stimulates the abdominal region. Be careful not to push or force any stage of this sequence. The full posture can make some people feel claustrophobic—so take it slowly if you are prone to this phobia.

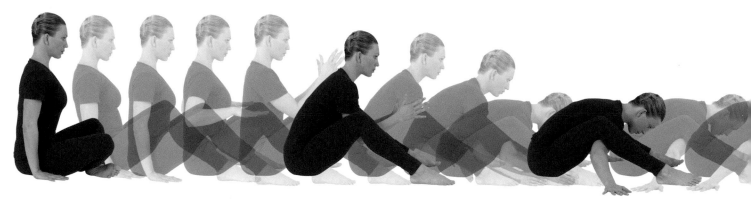

● Sit on the floor with your legs crossed together and the soles facing out to the sides. Place your hands on the floor either side of your bottom, and point the fingertips forward.

● Slowly uncross your legs and extend them in front of you. Place your feet on the floor, spacing them one and a half hip's width apart. Keep your knees bent.

● Leaning forward, bring your arms in front of you; then take them out to the sides, sliding them under your knees. Place your palms flat on the floor, with fingertips pointing outward.

● Lift your toes, keeping your heels on the floor. Inhale and lift your chest away from the hips.

▶ **inhale** ▶ **exhale** ▶ **inhale** ▶

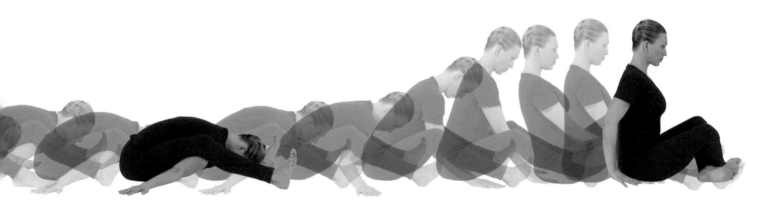

● Shuffle your heels forward as you lower your chest and chin. Slide your hands so that the fingertips point away from you. Press your legs against your upper arms, making sure not to press down on the elbows.

● If it feels comfortable, try lifting your heels off the floor. Hold this position for five breaths. This is known as the turtle *asana*.

● Release the position, placing your heels back on the floor and bringing your arms to the front. Slowly lift your chest upward and hold your head upright to look forward.

● Draw your legs into your body, with your feet crossed. Straighten the back and neck, and place your hands on the floor on either side of your bottom. Now perform the half *Vinyasa*.

exhale ❙❙ ▶ inhale exhale ❙❙

restrained angle *baddha konasana*

This *asana* is often described as the traditional pose of an Indian cobbler. It stimulates the blood supply to the pelvis, abdomen, and back, and is also an effective exercise for opening the hip.

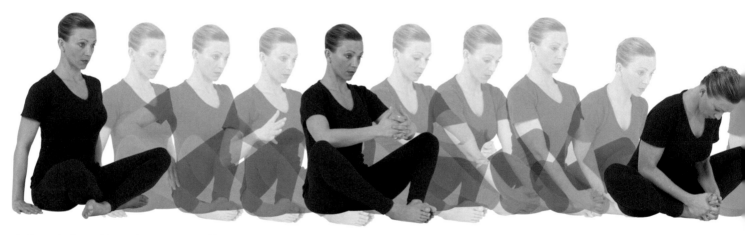

● Sit on the floor with your legs crossed together and the soles facing out to the sides. Place your hands on the floor either side of your bottom, and point the fingertips forward.

● Uncross your legs and bring the soles of your feet together. Lift up your hands and bring your arms to the front. Join the hands together, interlocking your fingers.

● Hook your clasped hands over both feet and gently pull them in toward your groin. Lift your chest upward and straighten your arms Hold this position for five breaths. Move your shoulders away from your ears.

● Tuck your chin in so that your neck is aligned with your spine. Slowly fold your body forward from your hips. Bend your arms into your sides and relax your knees toward the floor. Hold for five breaths.

exhale ▶ **inhale** ▶ **exhale**

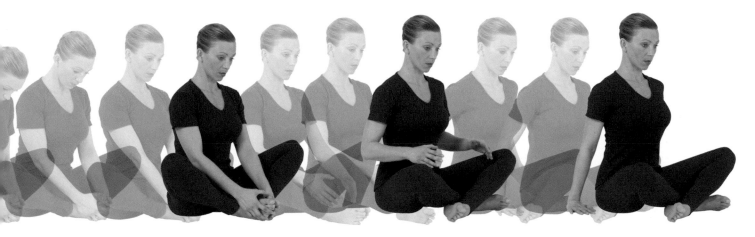

● Release the position. Still holding onto the feet, bring the torso upright and straighten your arms.

● Unlock your fingers and release your feet. Hold your head upright and straighten your spine.

● Raise your arms and take them behind you. Place your hands on the floor on either side of your bottom, with fingertips facing forward.

● Draw your legs into your body, with your feet crossed. Straighten the back and neck. Now perform the half *Vinyasa* before starting the next *asana*.

inhale ▶   **exhale** ▶   **inhale** ▶   **II**

seated angle

uparista konasana

This *asana* stretches your hamstrings and helps to increase flexibility in your hips. Make sure that the backs of your legs rest on the floor and the knees and toes point at the ceiling.

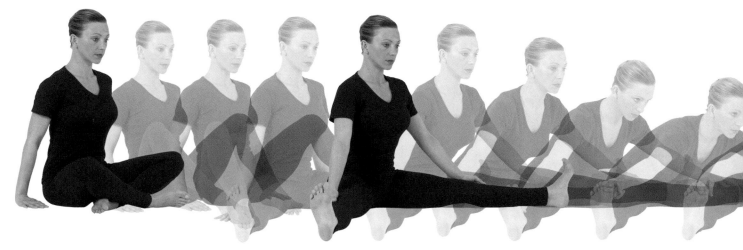

● Sit on the floor with your legs crossed in front of you and the soles of your feet facing out to the sides. Place your hands by your thighs, with palms pressed on the floor and fingertips pointing forward.

● Uncross your legs and extend them out to the side, keeping the spine straight and your toes and knees pointing up toward the sky.

● Raise your hands off the floor and rest them on your thighs. Lift your chest upward, and tuck your chin in.

● Slowly fold your body over, bending from the hips. Keep your neck and spine in line with each other.

inhale ▶ ▶ **exhale** ▶

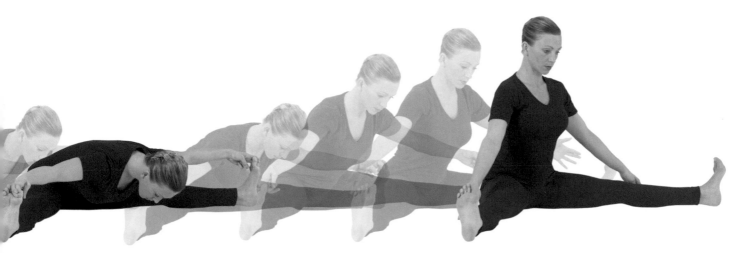

● Slide your hands along the length of your legs, and hook your big toes with the thumb and forefinger of each hand. Hold this position for five breaths.

● Release the position and slowly raise your chest away from the floor. Unhook your toes and rest your hands on your legs.

● Lift your body into the upright position, keeping your back straight. Hold your head upright and focus on a point in front of you.

● Bring your arms back to your sides, keeping your legs extended with your toes pointing upward. Continue into the next sequence without pausing.

II   **inhale**   ▶   **exhale**   ▶

lying down angle

supta konasana

You may find it more comfortable to hold your feet by the ankles; with time, you will

be able to progress to holding the toes for a more intense stretch.

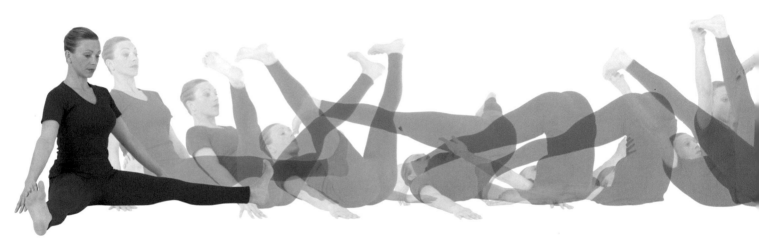

● Sit on the floor with your legs outstretched and spaced wide apart in front of you. Place your hands on the floor at either side of your bottom.

● Using your arms to support your body weight, slowly roll back onto your shoulders.

● Keeping your legs extended and spread apart, raise them up and over your head to the floor. Take the arms along the floor and hold your big toes. Hold this position for five breaths.

● As you raise your feet off the floor, pull against your feet to lift your upper body away from the floor. Balance with your spine straight.

exhale   ▶   exhale   ▶   inhale   ▶

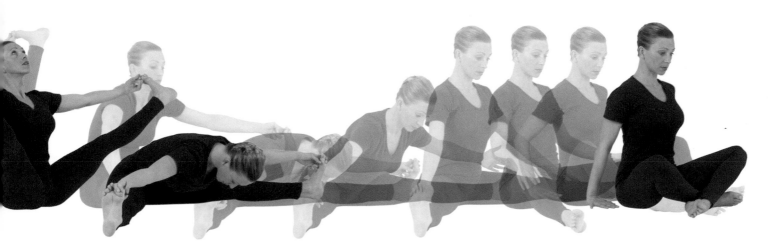

● Still holding the toes, fold forward, taking the legs down to the floor. Extend your torso down to the floor.

● Release your feet and slowly lift your chest away from the floor. Slide your arms back along your legs, and rest your hands on your knees.

● Draw your legs into your body with your feet crossed. Straighten the back and neck, and place your hands behind you with the fingers pointing forward.

● Push down into the floor with your hands. Now perform the half *Vinyasa* before starting the next *asana*.

exhale   inhale   ▶   inhale   ‖ exhale   ▶   ‖

finishing postures

arched bow *dhanurasana*

The focus of this movement is on the spine, which will become supple and strong with regular practice. This is a less challenging version of the Full Back Bend (pp 106–107). It opens the front of the body and tones the thighs. Keep your buttocks relaxed during this sequence.

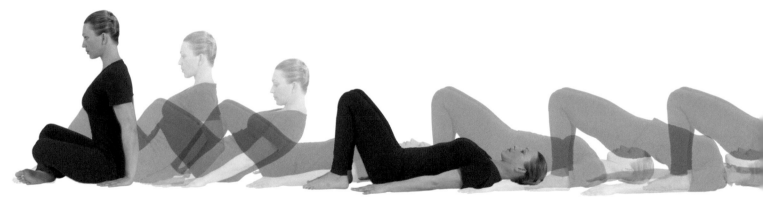

● Sit on the floor with your legs crossed in front of you and the soles of your feet facing out to the sides. Place your hands by your thighs, with palms pressed on the floor and fingertips pointing forward.

● Keeping your legs bent, uncross your feet and place them on the floor in front of the hips.

● Draw your feet closer to your bottom, so that your shins are vertical. Rest your extended arms by your sides, with palms facing downward.

● Press your hands against the floor as you push your hips and chest up toward the sky. Keep your feet firmly planted on the floor and parallel to each other. Slide your arms under your body and interlock the fingers.

exhale ▶ ▶ **inhale** ▶

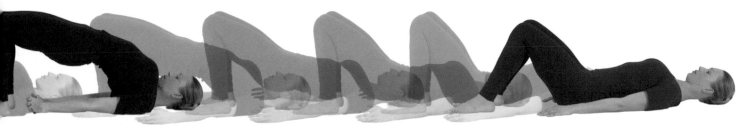

● Extend your arms toward your feet as your shoulders roll back and your chest moves higher. Use your feet and shoulders to push your body away from the floor. Hold this position for five breaths.

● Release the position by gently lowering your spine to the floor, working from the shoulders down to your bottom. Unclasp your hands and take your arms out to the sides with palms facing downward.

● Slide your legs away from your body, still keeping the knees bent and soles pressed against the floor.

● Straighten your back and neck, and relax your shoulders into the floor. Breathe deeply.

exhale ▶   inhale   **ll**

lying twist

counterpose to arched bow

When raising your knees and turning the body, try to keep your lower back on the floor, and lift only

from the hips. This sequence forms the counterpose to the previous *asana*.

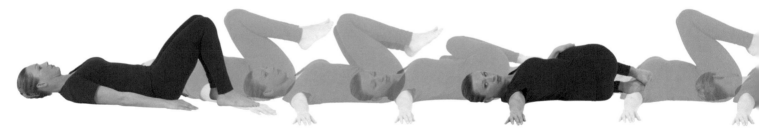

● Lie on the floor, with your shoulders relaxed and stomach pulled in. Rest your arms at the sides, with the fingertips pointing forward. Bend your legs and space your feet slightly apart from each other.

● Raise your feet off the floor and slowly bring your knees up toward your chest. Slide your arms across the floor and extend them out to the sides at shoulder height.

● Gently turn your head to look along your right arm. Pressing your palms into the floor, twist your knees and hips to the left side, and rest your knees on the floor. Check that your right shoulder stays on the floor.

● Release the position, taking your left arm out to the side at shoulder height. Slowly roll your knees and hips back to the center.

▶   **inhale**   ▶   **exhale**   ▶   **inhale**   ❚❚   ▶

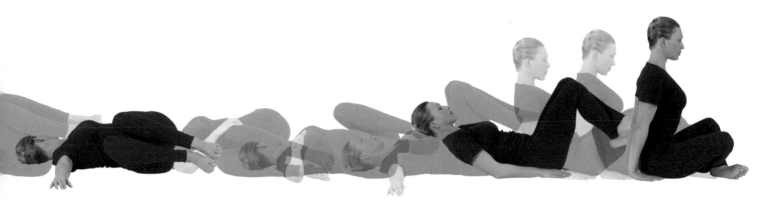

● Gently turn your head to look along your left arm. Pressing your palms into the floor, twist your knees and hips to the right side, and rest your knees on the floor. Check that your left shoulder stays on the floor.

● Release the position, taking your right arm out to the side at shoulder height. Slowly roll your knees and hips back to the center.

● Lower your feet to the floor, crossing your legs in mid air. Pressing your palms against the floor, push your body into the upright position and tuck your feet under your knees.

● Slide your hands behind you, either side of your bottom, with fingertips pointing forward.

exhale   inhale || exhale   ▶   inhale   ▶ ||

full back bend *urdhva dhanurasana*

The Full Back Bend opens the front of the body and has intense toning effects on the spine.

Check that your palms are spaced apart no more than shoulder width for the bend itself.

The squeezing effect detoxes the liver and kidneys, and may make some people feel light headed.

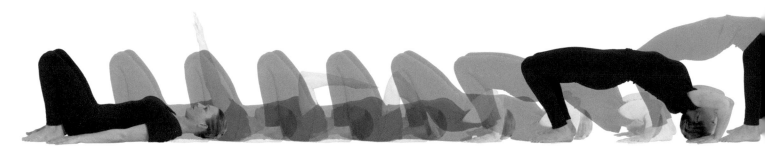

● Lie on the floor with your shoulders relaxed and stomach pulled in. Rest your arms at the sides, with the fingertips pointing forward. Bend your legs, keeping your shins vertical, and place your feet hip width apart.

● Slowly raise your extended arms in front of you; then take them above your head. With fingertips pointing toward you, press your palms on the floor underneath your shoulders.

● Pressing into the floor with feet and hands, push the chest and hips up to the ceiling, bringing the crown of the head to the floor between the hands.

● Continue pushing the chest and hips up so that your arms and legs are extended as far as possible. Let your head hang down so that the crown points toward the floor.

▶ **inhale**　　　　　▶　　　　　▶ **exhale**　　　　　▶

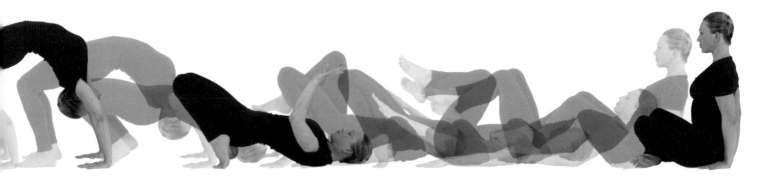

● Check that your feet are still parallel, and keep the soles pressed into the floor. Hold this position for five breaths.

● Release the position, slowly lowering your body toward the floor. As your shoulders touch the floor, take your hands off the floor and lift your arms over your head. Rest them on the floor at your sides.

● Raise your feet onto the toes to ease your bottom onto the floor; then lift your knees into the air and cross your feet over. Pressing your palms against the floor, push your body into the upright position.

● Tuck your feet under your knees and slide your hands to either side of your bottom, with fingertips pointing forward.

inhale ‖ exhale ▶   inhale ▶   ‖

forward bend counterpose
paschimottanasana

Having performed the Full Back Bend, it is good practice to follow the movement with a Forward

Bend as a counterpose as it refreshes the body after the intense stretch of the Full Back Bend.

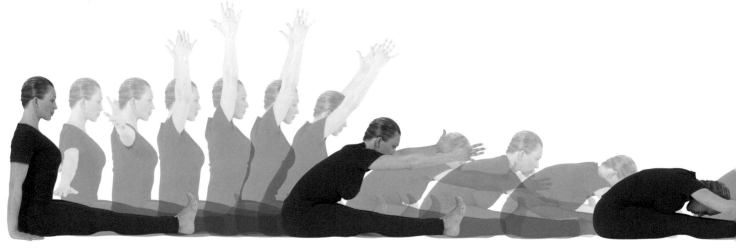

● Start in the Rod position, with your legs extended in front and toes pointing upward. Place your hands on the floor on either side of your bottom, and focus your eyes on a point in front of you.

● Keeping your neck and back straight, extend both arms in front of you and raise them overhead, with fingertips pointing upward.

● Slowly fold the body forward, moving your chest toward the knees. Keep your spine as straight as possible. Grasp the outside edges of your feet with both hands. Tuck your chin in and hold for five breaths.

● If this position does not feel comfortable, slide your hands to your ankles and hold them for five breaths.

inhale ▶ exhale ▶ ‖ ▶

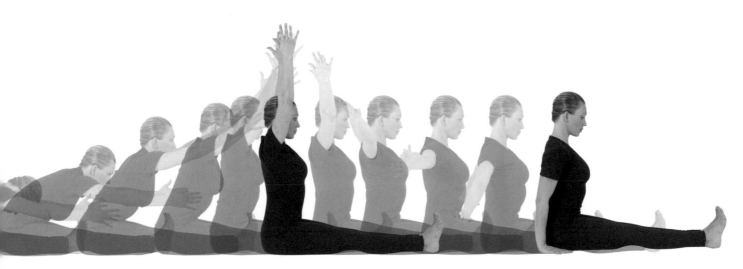

● Release the position. Slowly raise your body away from the ground, releasing your feet or ankles. Keep the toes pointing upward and heels resting on the ground.

● Take your extended arms above the head, focusing on keeping your neck and spine straight.

● Slowly lower the arms down to your sides, and position them on either side of your bottom, with palms pressed against the floor.

● Keep your back and neck straight and hold your head upright. Relax and breathe deeply. Now perform the half *Vinyasa* before the next *asana*.

inhale　▶　**exhale**　**11**

shoulder stand *sirsasana*

This movement is performed in two stages; intermediate students should start with the Half Shoulder Stand and progress to the Full Shoulder Stand once they feel confident and strong enough to hold the position. This sequence continues into the Plough on the next page.

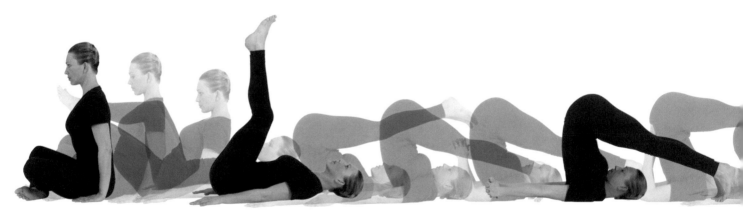

● Sit on the floor with your legs crossed in front of you and the soles of your feet facing out to the sides. Place your hands by your thighs, with palms pressed on the floor and fingertips pointing forward.

● Uncross your feet and extend your legs to the front, as you slowly lower your body toward the ground. Press into your palms to support your body and rest your elbows on the floor.

● Raise your legs upward then take them above your head and over the shoulders until your toes touch the floor behind you.

● Slide your arms in front you, keeping them extended, and clasp your hands together with interlocked fingers. Keep your back and legs straight and lift the top of the spine off the floor.

exhale   ▶   ▶   **inhale**   ▶

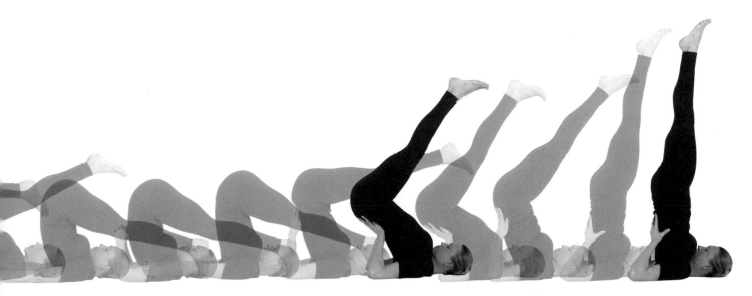

● Release your hands and place them at the top of your bottom. Raise your legs to a 90-degree angle to your body. Sit the weight of your bottom into the hands as you lift and open your chest.

● This is a Half Shoulder Stand—suitable for beginner and intermediate students. Hold the position for five breaths.

● For advanced students, push your feet toward the sky, using your hands to support your back. Slowly bring your shoulders, hips, and ankles into one straight line.

● Straighten your back, point your toes toward the sky, and tuck your chin into the chest. Hold the position for five breaths. Now go straight into the next *asana*, the Plough.

exhale ▶   ‖ **inhale** ▶   ‖ ▶

plough and ear press

balasana & karnapidasana

This movement progresses
from the Half and Full
Shoulder Stand. This
sequence can stimulate
the thyroid gland and so
should be avoided by anyone
with an overactive thyroid.

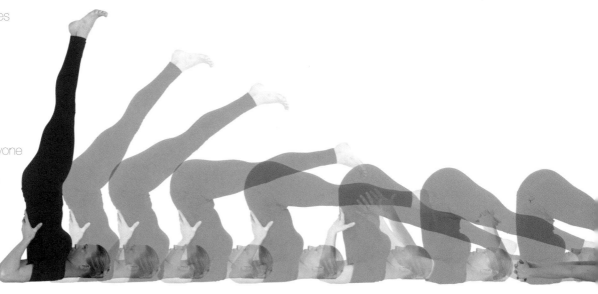

● From the Half and Full Shoulder Stand, slowly lower your extended legs over your head.

● Use your hands to support your lower back.

● As your feet come into contact with the floor, take your hands down to the floor. Try to keep your spine as straight as possible, and check that your hips remain directly in line with your shoulders.

● Slide your hands to the front and clasp them together. Hold the Plough position for five breaths.

▶ **exhale**   ▶ **inhale**   ▶ **exhale**   ▶

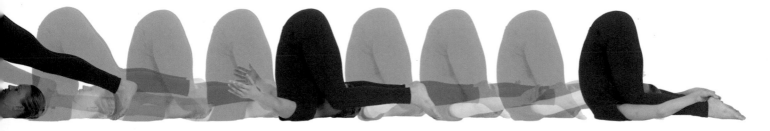

● Release the position and bend your legs to bring your knees down around your ears. Unclasp your hands and extend your arms out to the sides, keeping the shoulders on the floor.

● Keep your movements slow and steady during this sequence, and roll out of the pose if your feel any pain or discomfort in the neck or spine.

● Take your arms behind your head and over the calves of your legs. Place the palms of your hands on your heels, with fingertips pointing away from the body.

● Press your knees gently against your ears, and point your toes away from the body. Hold this position for five breaths. This sequence continues on the next page.

exhale ▶ ▶ ❚❚ ▶

plough and ear press *karnapidasana*

The second stage of this movement focuses on controlling the body as it unfurls. Concentrate on lowering the legs as slowly as possible, pausing whenever the movement starts to become jerky and strained. With practice you will achieve a smooth, flowing transition.

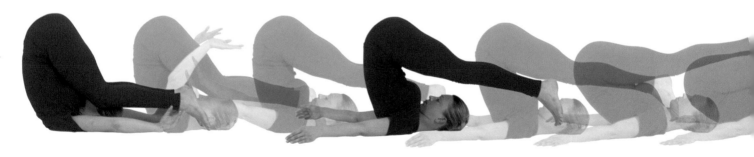

● Release the Ear Press position, raising your extended arms upward. Take them over your head and let them rest at your sides.

● Lift your knees off the floor and away from your ears. Keep your head and neck on the floor.

● Extend your legs fully, with toes pointing toward the floor. Slowly raise them above your head as you unfold your body from the hips.

● Lower your back one vertebra at a time, controlling the movement to make it a smooth, flowing transition.

▶   **inhale**   ▶   **exhale**   ▶   ▶

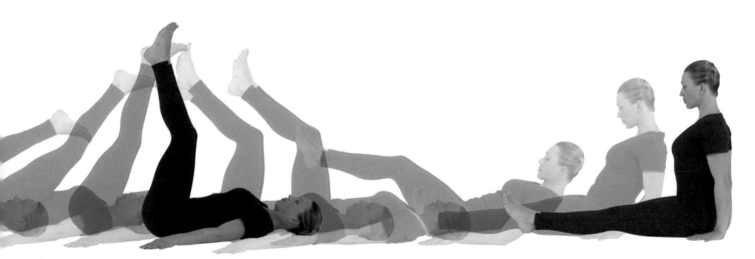

● As your bottom touches the floor, bend your legs slightly and bring the feet to the floor.

● Pressing the palms into the floor by your bottom, come to an upright sitting position.

● Slide your hands toward your bottom to support your body into the upright position.

● Assume the Rod position, with legs outstretched and toes pointing forward. Straighten your back and neck and hold your head upright. Continue into the next *asana*.

inhale ▶   ▶

fish *matsyasana*

The Fish *asana*, combined with the *Uttana Padasana*, enhance your breathing as they allow a full expansion of the chest. Stop the sequence if you feel any pain or discomfort in the spine.

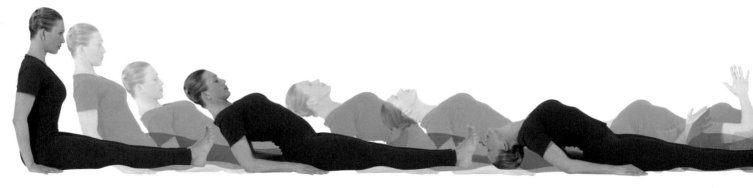

● Start in the Rod position, with your legs extended in front and toes pointing upward. Place your hands on the floor either side of your bottom, and focus your eyes on a point in front of you.

● Open your chest and lift the spine, creating an arch in your back. Bend your elbows and bring your forearms to rest on the floor. Focus your eyes on your toes.

● Maintaining the arch in your back, tilt your head back until the crown is resting on the floor. This is the Fish. Hold for five breaths. If it is too uncomfortable to rest on your head, support your weight with your elbows.

● If your head is on the floor, lift your hands off the floor and slowly raise your extended arms in front of you at an angle of 45 degrees.

▶   **inhale**   ▶   **exhale**   **‖ inhale**   ▶

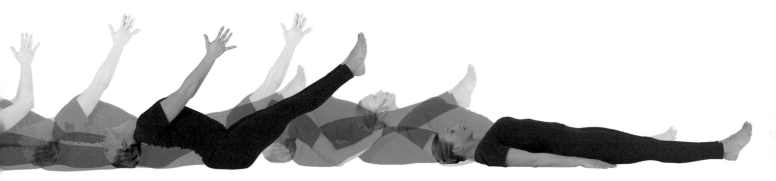

● Keeping your back arched and the crown of your head pressed into the floor, raise your extended legs to an angle of 45 degrees. Keep your arms and legs parallel to each other. This is *Uttana Padasana*. Hold for five breaths.

● Slowly release the position, lowering your legs toward the floor. Bring your arms down to your sides, pressing your elbows into the floor to support your back.

● Lift up your head and release the arch in your back. Relax your head, back, and shoulders into the floor.

● Rest your heels on the floor, with toes pointing forward. Settle the spine in its normal alignment.

exhale

headstand

There are two stages to the movement. The first stage allows the body to become balanced, and should be comfortable for you before you move to the next stage. The second stage takes you to the Full Headstand.

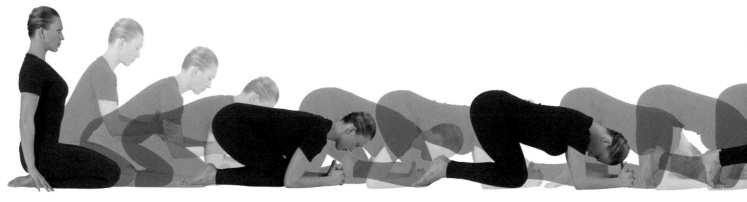

● Kneel on the floor with your feet tucked underneath your bottom. Hold your back and head upright, keeping your neck aligned with your spine. Place your arms at your sides, with fingertips resting on the floor.

● Slowly lean your body forward, bending from the hips. Bring your arms to the front and place your elbows on the floor, outside of your knees. Clasp your hands together, interlocking the fingers.

● Tilt your head toward the floor, tucking your chin into the chest. Keeping your elbows in line with your shoulders, gently shuffle your knees away from your body.

● Place the crown of your head on the floor, and cradle the back of your head with your hands.

■ inhale   exhale   ▶   ▶   inhale   ▶

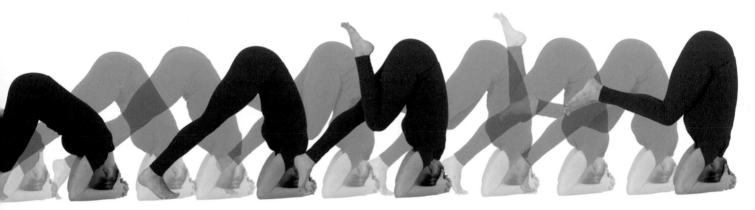

● Raise your feet onto your toes and press against the floor to straighten your legs. Gently push your body into an inverted "V" shape.

● Keep your shoulders away from your ears, and make sure that your body weight is supported by your shoulders and arms, not your neck.

● Walk your feet as close to your body as is comfortable. Slowly raise your right heel to your bottom as you bring your right knee into your chest. Hold this position for a few breaths.

● Release your right foot from the upright position and slowly lower it to the floor. Repeat this position on the left leg and hold for a few breaths. This sequence continues on the next page.

exhale   **inhale**   **II**   **exhale**   ▶   **II** ▶   ▶

headstand *sirsasana*

Approach the headstand with confidence, rather than fear, and you will achieve the position with ease. You may feel light headed after this *asana* so take it easy.

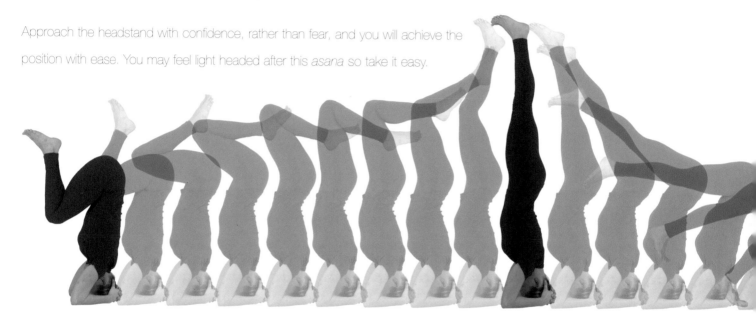

● You are now ready to move into the full headstand position. Slowly raise the heels to your bottom and your knees into your chest.

● Check that your body weight is supported by the arms and shoulders. Start taking the knees toward the sky. Open the front of the body as your knees come up.

● Slowly unfold the legs, taking the feet toward the sky until your body forms a vertical line. Hold the position for five breaths—or longer if you find it comfortable.

● Release the position, slowly lowering your extended legs until your toes touch the floor. Keep the movement slow and controlled.

▶ **exhale**   **inhale** ▶   ● **exhale** ▶

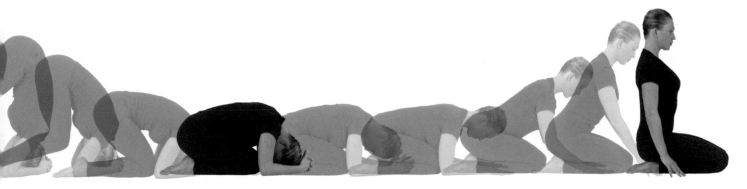

● Bend your knees and bring them into your chest. Lower your bottom down toward your heels, bringing it to rest on your shins.

● Slowly lift your head away from the floor, and release your clasped hands. Place your palms face down on the floor in front of you.

● Keeping your neck in line with your spine, lift your body into the upright position. Raise your arms off the floor and bring them in to your sides, with fingertips pointing downward.

● Resume the kneeling position with feet tucked under your bottom, chest lifted, and head facing forward.

inhale   exhale   ▶   inhale   ▶   ‖

child's pose into gentle neck stretch

The stretch felt in your neck should be very gentle and gradual; if it feels

painful or uncomfortable at any time, release the position and relax.

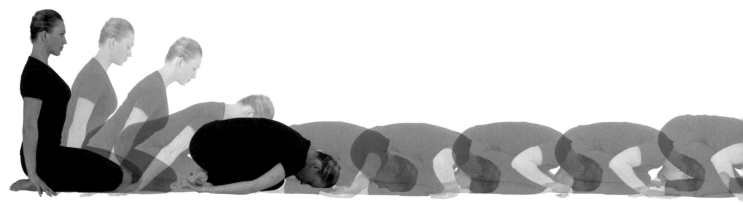

● Kneel on the floor with your feet tucked underneath your bottom. Hold your back and head upright, keeping your neck aligned with your spine. Place your arms at your sides, with fingertips resting on the floor.

● Slowly lean your body forward, bending from the hips. Bring your forehead to rest on the floor and slide your hands by your feet with the backs of the hands on the floor.

● Rest your chest against your thighs and hold the position for five breaths—or longer if desired. This is the Child's pose.

● Release the position and bring your hands forward. Place your palms on the floor in front of the knees and shoulder width apart.

▶   **exhale**   ▶   **inhale**   ▶

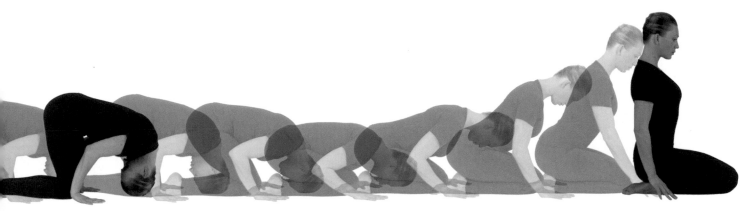

● Pressing your hands against the floor, lift your bottom upward and roll softly over your head. Keep your shoulders away from your ears.

● Roll back onto your forehead. Repeat this movement three times to feel a gentle stretch in your neck.

● Press your palms into the floor, and slowly lift your chest away from your thighs. Keep the neck and back aligned as you return to the upright position.

● Straighten your back and hold your head upright. Focus on a point ahead of you. Rest your arms at your sides, with fingertips resting on the floor by your heels. Relax and breathe.

exhale   **inhale**   ▶   **exhale**   ▶   **II**

lotus and corpse *padmasana, tolasana, & savasana*

If the Lotus position below puts any pressure on your knees or hips, simply cross your legs instead.

It is easy to hurt yourself in this posture if you are not careful, so be patient and take it easy. The

Corpse should be practiced at the end of every session as it allows your body to rest and relax,

giving you the chance to recuperate and feel refreshed, not exhausted.

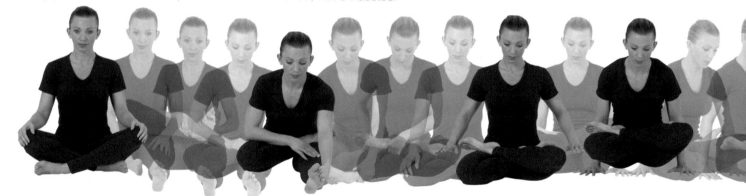

● Sit on the floor with your legs crossed in front of you and the soles of your feet facing out to the sides. Place your hands on your knees, and focus your eyes on a point in front of you. Keep your shoulders relaxed.

● Tuck in your chin slightly so your neck is aligned with your spine. Uncross your legs and rest your right foot on top of your left thigh, with the sole facing upward and the heel pushing against the lower abdomen.

● Extend your left leg and fold forward from the hips to take hold of your left ankle with your left hand. Bring the left foot onto the right thigh, sole upward. Hold for about 20 breaths, hands resting on your knees.

● Place your hands on the floor, on either side of your bottom. Transfer your body weight onto your hands, and push into the floor to lift your bottom off the floor. Hold the position for as long as is comfortable.

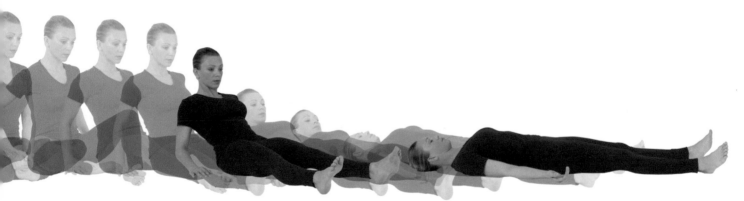

● Release the position, lowering your bottom to the floor. Slide your hands forward to take hold of your feet and unfold them.

● Place your hands on the floor, on either side of your bottom, and slowly lean your body back. Support your body with your forearms, bringing it to rest on the floor.

● Extend your legs, with toes pointing forward, and bring your arms down to your sides, with palms upward. Relax your shoulders and align your neck with your spine.

● Close your eyes, soften your body completely, and release any tensions. This is the Corpse *asana*. Relax and let go. Stay here for at least five minutes, longer if possible.

inhale   exhale   ▶   inhale   II

index

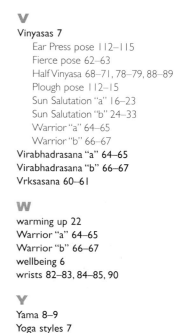

Author's Dedication
Dedicated with love to the memory
of Tony Duncan my guardian angel
who died on the 28 Nov 2001